SAGE
A MAN'S GUIDE INTO HIS SECOND PASSAGE

CHRIS BRUNO

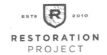

Copyright © 2022 by Chris Bruno

All rights reserved.

Except for brief quotations in critical publications or reviews, no part of this book may be reproduced, or stored in a retrieval system, or transmitted in any form or by any means, electronic, mechanical, photocopying, recording, or otherwise, without express written permission of the publisher.

Restoration Project

155 West Harvard St, STE 401

Fort Collins, CO 80525

ISBN-13: 979-8-218-01085-0

Cover design by: Cody Buriff, www.pinwheelcreative.net

All Scripture quotations, unless otherwise indicated, are taken from the Holy Bible, New International Version®, NIV®. Copyright ©1973, 1978, 1984, 2011 by Biblica, Inc.™ Used by permission of Zondervan. All rights reserved worldwide. www.zondervan.comThe "NIV" and "New International Version" are trademarks registered in the United States Patent and Trademark Office by Biblica, Inc.™

Scripture quotations taken from the (NASB®) New American Standard Bible®, Copyright © 1960, 1971, 1977, 1995, 2020 by The Lockman Foundation. Used by permission. All rights reserved. www.lockman.org

Scripture quotations marked "Darby" are taken from the Darby Translation Bible (Public Domain).

ENDORSEMENTS

The game of life, like any game, is about making halftime adjustments. Of course, it sure helps to have a coach like Chris Bruno. This book is a playbook. Thanks to Chris for sharing both his wit and wisdom. If you have the courage to apply these time-tested principles, the best is yet to come!
    Mark Batterson, Lead Pastor of National Community Church; New York Times Bestselling author of *The Circle Maker*

Most people either fail to dream of being a Sage or assume it is beyond the grasp of mere mortals. Chris Bruno, a wise, kind, and humble man, has invited us to walk with wisdom as we return to our younger selves, blessing the hardships and losses that have formed us as men. Chris offers a North Star vision of how a man becomes a Sage. You will find this brilliant book a trustworthy compass to guide you through the wilds of aging.
    Dan B. Allender. Ph.D, Professor of Counseling Psychology, The Seattle School of Theology and Psychology; Author of *Redeeming Heartache*

There are painfully few soul-strengthening messages that help the heart of a man finish well. We live in a world with many old men, but few sages, few men whose entire personhood is so drenched in maturity and wholeheartedness that they are capable of guiding the next generations to the farthest reaches of our masculine journey with wisdom and strength. In Chris Bruno, we have such a man. Curated with clarity and care, brimming with authentic stories of masculine initiation, and girded by courageous self-disclosure from Chris's own journey, Sage offers a trustworthy, God-shaped, timely message for men who deeply desire to experience the full portion of masculine maturity, build an enduring legacy in the second half of life, and finish well.

Morgan Snyder, Author of *Becoming a King;* Founder, www.BecomeGoodSoil.com; Vice President, Wild At Heart

This book was made possible by a generous grant from the Michael Cameron Dempsey Fund.

Michael's legacy is one of healing broken spaces in order to cultivate relationship among brothers who laugh, play, create, and know God. After his too-soon passing, his family has committed to making his memory evergreen.

May this work both honor his life and his legacy for years to come.

CONTENTS

Introduction — ix

PART ONE
A VISION FOR THE SECOND HALF

1. Meeting Gandalf, the Hero's Hero — 3
2. The Masculine Destination — 13

PART TWO
THE FIRST HALF

3. The Divine Masterpiece — 27
4. The First Passage of a Man's Life — 41
5. The Man of the First Half — 49
6. Failed Projections — 59
7. Personas: The Masks We Wear — 72
8. Midlife — 82
9. Coming to the End of Ourselves — 92

PART THREE
THE SAGE OF THE SECOND HALF

10. The Sage's Enough: Settled Contentment — 113
11. The Sage's Welcome: A Spacious Inner Hospitality — 125
12. The Sage's Great God: Generous Spirituality — 137
13. The Sage's Death: The Crucible of Suffering — 146
14. The Sage's Companion: From Loneliness to Solitude — 159
15. The Sage's Boy: Bringing Him Home — 173

Conclusion	193
Acknowledgments	199
Bibliography	203
Notes	209
About the Author	219
Restoration Project	221
Restoration Counseling	223
Introduction to Brotherhood Primer	225

INTRODUCTION

The subterranean tremors began to shake our lives in ways we did not understand. We felt the tectonic shifts deep within and somehow recognized the call to a new adventure, a new season, a new exploration of our lives as men. When we were younger, we may have understood this as a beckoning towards a higher mountain to climb, a steeper slope to ski, a more impossible business to start, or a greater promotion to attain. But now, each of us in midlife, we knew this was altogether different. This call took us to the Scottish Highlands.

Something psychological happens in a man's life when he crosses the 40-year-old threshold. He wakes up to his limitations with a keen awareness that the morning of his life will soon turn towards afternoon. There is just as much behind as there is ahead, and he must reckon with the fact that midlife has arrived. The passage into a new season is about to begin.

There are two such passages in a man's life: first, when he transforms from boy into man; and second, when that same man transforms into Sage. These kinds of thresholds must be marked, celebrated, and remembered. As John O'Donohue writes, "A threshold is not a simple boundary; it is a frontier that divides two different territories, rhythms, and atmospheres."[1] Choosing to live as intentional fathers, the men on this Scottish adventure had already been journeying together with our sons' rites of passage we came to call the *Man Maker Project*.[2] We had been attending to the hearts of our boys, crafting intentional experiences, exploring Godly characteristics of manhood, and inviting them to deeper relationships with other adult men, seeking to answer their core questions, *"Am I a man? Do I have what it takes?"* with a resounding *"Yes!"* And while our boys were in various stages of their first passage, we all knew boys do not instantly become men. All passages take years. We all know, years matter.

But for the four of us men, as our soul-tremors grew louder and stronger and more insistent, we found *ourselves* at a new threshold of manhood, a second passage, one we knew we needed to cross. This next journey would require an equal amount of ritual, intention, and reflection. And so, together with three of my closest friends, Greg, Bart, and Shae, we set out on an epic pilgrimage to Scotland in search of our own selves.

At Restoration Project, we believe the three core conditions of life-changing moments are *experience, story,* and *blessing*.[3] Therefore, Greg and I partnered to craft a meaningful journey pairing physical adventure with soulful content. As a result, we canoed, kayaked, hiked, and toured distillery after distillery, all while inviting reflection, story, and mutual pursuit of each other's hearts. And while it began with a once-in-a-lifetime journey to the Scottish Highlands, the crossing of the spiritual and psychological threshold continues for each of us even years later. Just as ushering a boy into manhood takes intention, so too the passage of a man into the Sage requires purpose and focus. Most men, however, go on living their lives without an awareness of their own deep need for this intentional work. It is our second passage into manhood, into the second half, that far too many men resist, neglect, or deny.

As a therapist[4] and leader of a men's ministry organization,[5] I have spent countless hours with men at all stages of the masculine journey: adolescent boys who long for a father to lead them, notice them, and bless them for who they are and not what they do; young men in their 20s first embracing the vigor of their lives as men as they pursue work and women, pushing the limits of their daring and power; guys in their 30s, grappling with increased responsibility at home and work, facing what it means to be faithful husband, intentional father, and adult son; men in their 40s and 50s, wondering what life is really about, realizing the prescribed formulas of the world and church do not always yield the promised results; and men in their 60s, 70s and 80s, who find themselves regretful, lonely, and pining for days gone by. With each of these men, I witnessed a deep inner struggle to orient themselves in the man-life God has given them. We must consider manhood as a journey, not a destination. Often, I ask men, "When did you become a man?" Answers to this question are all over the map, including "when I left home" or "when I got my first job" or "when I had sex for the first time" or "when I got my driver's license" or "when I became a father." Again, no one has ever said, "I'm still becoming a man." The fact is, we are all still becoming men because we are still discovering the mystery of who God made us to be and why. The manhood journey is cyclical rather than linear, and the further along we travel, we find ourselves once again at the beginning, calling "us both backward and forward, to our foundation and our future, at the same time."[6] To cross the second threshold from man into Sage, we must be prepared to go deeper and in reverse to recover those parts of us we exiled, forgot, lost, or never fully knew.

There are four primary movements in a man's life: (1) when he is born, (2) when he crosses the threshold from boy to man, (3) when he recovers his True Self and crosses the threshold to the second half, and (4) when he dies. We have very little influence on our own physical beginning and ending. Birth and death are ruled by forces beyond us (though we do everything we can to gain God-like control). The two movements in which we consciously and purposefully participate are crossing of the two thresholds: the passages from boy to man and from man to Sage. While I have written about the first passage elsewhere,[7] my task here is to explore the depths and challenges of the second passage and what it means to enter and thrive in the second half.

If the task of the first passage is to find the man within the boy and call him forth, the task of the second passage is to find the boy within the man and bring him home.

THE PATH

I have divided this work into three main parts:

In Part 1, I set forth a vision for the Sage, exploring God's purposes for this second passage, and the men he designed us to become. We consider the devastating impact our world experiences when men merely grow old without becoming Sages, and we reflect on the biblical understanding of "elder." We survey history and culture to understand the Sage as the pinnacle of God's masculine design. In this section, we will answer the question, "Why is the transformation from man into Sage both vital and biblical?"

In Part 2, we explore the vital segments of a man's first half, uncovering the important stages through which a man must pass before he can cross the threshold of the second half. We rediscover the divine masterpiece written into the narrative of our lives and discuss the first passage from boy to man. I help you identify your *projections* and your *personas*, two ways we survive our first half that cannot accompany us across the second threshold. We explore the shaky ground of midlife, and then, we conclude by recognizing the importance of coming to the end of ourselves before we take the first steps into the second half. In this section, we will answer the questions, "What is the first half, and what does a man do to prepare himself for the second?"

In Part 3, we explore the six hallmark characteristics of the Sage, including settled contentment, spacious inner hospitality, generous spirituality, the crucible of suffering, and the move from loneliness to solitude. We end with the culmination of the journey as the Sage welcomes back his younger lost self, returning the boy to the man. In this section, we will explore the questions, "What makes a man a Sage, and how does one navigate the transition over the threshold of the second passage to become his True Self?"

DISCLOSURES AND WARNINGS

Throughout each section, I share a variety of stories. To protect confidentiality, I have changed names and details in an attempt to honor the stories and hard soul-work of the many brave men with whom I have had the privilege of journeying into some of their darkest and most vulnerable places. In fact, while everything I have written is true, all stories are an amalgamation of many. We come to know our own stories through the stories of others, and as such, it is my hope you will find yourself in the stories shared. Should one of them strike close to home, I invite you to deepen your curiosity about what God may have for you there.

While I have a deep love and respect for women, and I believe women could benefit from what I offer here, my primary audience is men. Certainly, there are many similarities between men and women when it comes to the first and second halves of our lives. However, as a man and as a leader of men's work, it is my focus and task to come alongside women in the *recovery* of their men. When we recognize the unique value God has placed on humanity *as men* and *as women*, we discover a more complete understanding of God's image. May the words here provide nourishment for whoever finds them.

Personally, I am on the front end of this life transition. Though the epic journey to Scotland took place years ago, as I sit today and write, I am a young 49 years old. I do not have the experience and tenure of my 60s, 70s, or 80s. The voices of these older sages ring loudly in my ears, and I cherish their thoughts, words, and wisdom both for this work and for my own journey.[8] I have always endeavored to live life out loud, to share my reflections and experiences *as they occur* with men I consider my contemporaries. My hope is to give words to the crucible men face in our middle years, our first steps into the second half, and to offer hope and direction.

As an ordained minister and a licensed therapist, I find the streams of both theology and psychology to be filled with refreshing waters, complementary in their insights, and suitable for guidance and soul care. As a follower of Jesus, I look to him for life and existence and sustenance. Nothing exists, even myself, without the benevolent generosity of the Creator. I exist because he does.

MY JOURNEY TO IRELAND

Knowing a pilgrimage is a "physical journey with a spiritual destination," to write this book I have once again embarked on an epic expedition, this time to the far western coast of Ireland. In January. *Alone.*

I sit within feet of the most westerly shores of Europe, coastlines where the rage of the winter sea breaks violently and constantly against the rugged cliffs of this ancient Celtic island. Rain is a forever companion here, and the crackle of the fire a constant reminder of God's warming presence. Whereas I came to the Isles several years ago with friends, this time I knew I needed to come by myself. No one can help me recover my boy, the ultimate mission of the second-half Sage. That is my aim, and I must do it alone. And as you will see, it is the charge of every second-half man to find those parts of himself he lost long, long ago. While not every man can or should plan a trip such as this, throughout these pages I invite you to join me on my spiritual journey as it coincides with my physical one.

As G.K. Chesterton says, "We are all under the same mental calamity; we have all forgotten our names. We have all forgotten what we really are."[9] On this journey into the second half, let us answer the call to remember our God-given identity, purpose, and meaning.

Let's bring our boys home.

PART ONE
A VISION FOR THE SECOND HALF

1

MEETING GANDALF, THE HERO'S HERO

My foot rested on the split rail as we leaned against the fence every Tuesday and Thursday evening at dusk. His face rarely turned directly towards me; instead, he fixed his eyes resolutely on the view of the mountain range that called to something deep within us both. Though he said very few words, the corners of his mouth were always turned slightly upwards, as if gladness and peace lingered just below the surface of his weather-aged face. The arrangement had been made, an agreement never spoken but fully known: if I brought him coffee, I could stand there with him for as long as it took to drink.

My world had recently turned inside out, having just returned from a year-long student exchange in Germany as a junior in high school. It had been a flight of survival, getting away from the chaos of my home in a manner I convinced my parents would be "educational." Though I had no way to know this before I left, it was also the year the Eastern European block fell, and the divided continent launched into a celebratory yet tumultuous reunion. I lived 30 kilometers from the East German border, a border that dissolved while I watched nearby.

I left as a boy but came home a young man, the world and all its possibilities opened before me. Now a senior in high school, back in my small mountain hometown, the expansiveness of my heart simply could not be contained. Somehow, though, the man I stood next to at the fence knew it. He read it in me, and twice a week, he availed himself to bear witness to the rising tempest within me that refused to conform to my family's highly structured ways or my high school culture's infatuation with homecoming court. And so, we stood there, evening after evening, coffees in hand, in the liminal space between day and night and all the space I found so generously in his presence.

I knew Ben before I left on my international voyage. He served as the Young Life director for our rural mountain area even though he and his lovely wife, Judy, did not fit the typical caricature of what one imagines of a youth leader. They were older with a few children already raised and launched. This work with high schoolers was now their third career, the most recent having owned and operated an outdoor gear supply store. But Ben's dry and often surprising wit combined with his settled and spacious presence drew me in to want all I could get of him.

In my own home, I did not know this kind of presence. I did not know what it felt like to be near a solid and yet kind man. I knew a good man–loyal and generous and always providing for the physical needs of his family–but I did not know what it felt like to be safe, free, welcomed, and most of all, *with*. I grew up plotting my escape. Though violence and physical abuse are not part of my story, I learned early how to find emotional safety by disappearing from my father's presence. And so, twice a week on evenings before Young Life gatherings, I would show up early with coffees in hand, knowing that for a few moments I could absorb the goodness of a man who needed nothing from me but had everything to offer.

Roughly two decades later, I met another man like Ben. After living a lot of life, I was graciously and divinely introduced to Craig. Twenty years my senior, Craig had walked many of the same roads, and I found my heart often resonating with him. Though he lived two hours away, I did what I could to meet up with him when time and schedule allowed.

In the midst of a particularly troubling time, as I faced the mental and physical decline of my mother, the simultaneously increasingly challenging relationship with my father, and a stressful season of ministry, I reached out to Craig. He offered for me to come and spend the day with him at his house. No agenda, just come. It could have been a day of swapping stories, solving problems, giving advice, and plotting a way forward; instead, he offered me a *withness* that put my weary and troubled heart at ease. Craig generously asked questions, not for the sake of gathering information, but rather to open up my soul to receive the space and hospitality only another man could offer. He reminded me of God's goodness, kindness, and care. He blessed me and showed me the strong tenderness of a Sage that did not exist anywhere else in my life. I drove the two hours home that evening weeping, thanking God, and saying to myself, "I just met Gandalf."

I have talked with thousands of older men in my life—men who are further down the road in marriage, career, family, aging parents... you name it. I have sought counsel from many of them and have indeed received good advice along the way. But of the many older men with whom I have engaged, only a handful have been like Ben or Craig. There is something fundamentally different about these men, something that caused me to settle inside just by being in their presence. Only on a rare occasion will you meet an older man like this. Many are the gray-haired men who offer advice, mentoring, expertise, teaching, and discipleship. Many also are those who check out and fly south, living off the proceeds of their hard-won retirement funds, spending their days perfecting their golf swing and confirming their cruise ship plans. And many are those who have labored and waited for the days of retirement to truly live, sadly only to find their bodies no longer work or their minds are no longer sharp enough to manage.

But a few—just a few—of these older men have somehow found their way to a second half of life that offers a very needed Sage presence in the world. These remarkable men, these Sages, have the ability to stand next to a turbulent teen at a split-rail fence or welcome a middle-aged man into his living room and invite him to put down his sword and take off his armor to just *be*.

I believe God has a bigger vision for men and is calling the next several generations of men to step intentionally into the second half of their lives ready to further their presence rather than retreat; to bring a holy hospitality to the world in a way that invites and welcomes hearts to be and grow and become; and to stand as bastions of hope for the Kingdom to come even in the midst of our world's increased chaos and division. I believe the world needs more Gandalfs, Bens, and Craigs, and I intend to be among them. Will you join me?

THE FULL SPECTRUM OF MANHOOD AND THE MIDLIFE EARTHQUAKE

When most of us think about the seasons of a man's life, we generally imagine three main categories: (1) boy, (2) man, and (3) old man. "Boy" extends from birth to about 18 years old. At the other end of life, most people generally think the "old man" season starts at retirement age, today commonly considered as 65 years old and older. This leaves the "man" stage reaching from age 18 to age 65, a staggering 47-year span of life.

- Boy – between 0-18 years = 18 years of life
- Man – between 18-65 years = 47 years of life
- Old man – after 65 years = ~0-15 years[1]

But something happens in a man's life somewhere in his mid-30s and 40s, when he wakes up to the reality that the life he has lived so far may not be the life for which he is made. Those subterranean tremors deep within begin to shake, and as he stands at the halfway mark between birth and death, questions begin to rise to the surface. "Where am I going? What am I doing? What have I accomplished? Is this all there is? Another 25 to 30 years of *this* is what I have to look forward to?" All of these questions can be summarized into one: "What does my life even mean?"

In the foreword to psychiatrist and concentration camp survivor Viktor Frankl's book, *Man's Search for Meaning*, Harold Kushner wisely warns us, "Life is not primarily a quest for pleasure...or a quest for power...but a quest for meaning. The greatest task for any person is to find meaning in his or her life."[2] At the end of our days, we want to look back down the corridors of our lives and know the time God gave us on this earth meant something.

And so, somewhere in the middle of this 47-year journey between "boy" and "old man," we find ourselves in the middle of the middle. It is this nowhere-land between young and old, where we are neither yet both at the same time. It's unnerving and confusing, and we have very little guidance on how to pass over the next threshold into what many call the "second adulthood." Just as a boy must take the intentional and brave steps out of childhood and into manhood through a passage process, so too a middle-aged man must pass over a second threshold to enter the next season of his masculine journey. In the tumult of this middle space, a man must make a choice: to deny it and attempt to contain the stirrings within, to eject from his life in hopes of finding a better one elsewhere, or to set his jaw and engage the journey God has in store.

> In the tumult of this middle space, a man must make a choice: to deny it and attempt to contain the stirrings within, to eject from his life in hopes of finding a better one elsewhere, or to set his jaw and engage the journey God has in store.

James Hollis says it this way: "The experience...is not unlike awakening to find that one is alone on a pitching ship, with no port in sight. One can only go back to sleep, jump ship, or grab the wheel and sail on."[3]

Every middle-aged man has the opportunity to choose how to engage this next season of his life. Far too many men ignore the tremors of their soul, lulling themselves unconscious to the sweet promise of retirement. Others cannot take the pressure or disappointment, choosing instead to throw a grenade on their lives, blowing up their careers and families, convinced a new job, woman, or expensive toy will fill the void in their souls. But there are some, too few, who follow the wisdom of the ages and pursue their hearts, engage their questions, and follow God's leading into the Sage. The outcome of this choice is striking and significant: "Those who travel the passage consciously render their lives more meaningful. Those who do not, remain prisoners of childhood, however successful they may appear in outer life."[4] If a man does not engage, he will forever remain unfinished. Clearly, if we truly want our lives to be meaningful, we must turn towards the second-half threshold, not away, and wonder what treasures God may yet have buried for us in the inner territory of our masculine souls.

Maybe you have met your own Ben or Craig. I hope you have. You know who they are in your story—the Sages who have offered you their kindness, their presence, their acceptance, and their *withness*. Maybe you are one of the fortunates to have a man like this regularly in your life. Or perhaps you have only rubbed shoulders with this type of man once or twice. Still, I consider that lucky. Or, like many men, the Sages you know have long since passed from this earth, leaving a legacy in their words, thoughts, ideals, and manhood models for us to imitate. The fact is, none of these Sages simply woke up one day with wisdom, settledness, or presence. Their soul-level groundedness, their internal hospitality, and their generous grace resulted from hard-won battles against their own inner shadows in order to grow into a Sage.

THE OTHER HERO IN EVERY HERO'S JOURNEY

Think about the stories that capture your masculine imagination—the tales that have lodged themselves into your psyche as quintessential "man stories" and that you regularly revisit when you need hope, inspiration, or courage for your life. Or consider this: what are the legendary movies every young man should watch on his journey to become a man? When I've asked this question of men, the following movies top the list without fail: *Gladiator, The Lord of the Rings, Braveheart, The Last of the Mohicans, Star Wars,* even *Harry Potter.* Of course, there are many others, but these films are always on the list. Previous generations had a similar list, though possibly different storytelling forms, as narratives such as these have been told amongst men for millennia.

In each of these stories, we find a man in an epic battle against the forces of darkness and evil. Following the script Joseph Campbell named "the hero's journey," we see a familiar pattern:[5] the hero is called out of his ordinary life into an adventure; he originally refuses the call but then succumbs due to the magnitude of the need; as he starts out, he meets a mentor or guide along the way to offer him not only wisdom or insight, but also courage and heart for the journey; the hero embarks, leaving the safety of what is known, and starts down the road of peril; the hero fights battles, faces evil, and almost gives up before remembering the words of his guide, which reinvigorate his quest to vanquish the foe and win the day.

We know and love this storyline. We never tire of consuming these types of tales. And while most of the time, our focus (appropriately so) is on the hero and all he endures to win the war against evil, I want to draw your attention to the hero *behind* the hero. In each of these stories stands another important and powerful individual who shapes the trajectory of the narrative, and without whom, the story would not be a story.

- Who is Frodo or Aragorn without Gandalf?

- Who is Luke Skywalker without Yoda?
- Who is Maximus without Marcus Arelius?
- Who is Harry Potter without Albus Dumbledore?

In every epic tale we find a Sage at a critical crossroads of the hero's life. It is a ubiquitous element of all stories, across time and across cultures. Campbell's "monomyth" identifies a vital aspect of life's narrative: heroes only become heroes because the Sage is there to guide them.

The biblical narrative is no different. Sages fill the pages of the scripture and shape the course of the gospel story right from the beginning. We would not have the epic hero stories of the Christian faith if these heroes did not have the wisdom of a mature and present guide.

- Who was Samuel without Eli?
- Who was Moses without Jethro?
- Who was David without Nathan?
- Who was Timothy without Paul?

The stories of heroes are shaped by important Sages. From them, heroes draw wisdom, courage, clarity, strength, and power. These younger men[6] setting out on their ultimate quests must consult with an older guide to find the right path, obtain the magic potion, acquire the necessary weapon, or gain the secret wisdom to vanquish darkness. The journey does not become a *hero's journey* until he consults the Sage, for without him, he cannot become a hero.

And yet, how often do we pause long enough in our enjoyment of these tales to consider the Sage in the story? We are so transfixed by the warriors and the kings, the battles and the realms, the climactic moment when the hero vanquishes the villain, we neglect one of the most important individuals in the plotline. Yes, though we may know their names and nod our heads in gratitude for their part in the unfolding drama, the praise falls squarely with the hero. And often, especially in biblical narratives, we might not even know the name of the Sage at all.

During my son Aidan's "Man Year,"[7] he and I intentionally watched many of these classic "man movies" as both a welcome to manhood and an indoctrination into the character of men. I wanted him to see the hero's journey unfold on-screen, and then we discussed it together in the following weeks. We both loved this experience and bonded deeply, especially over *The Lord of the Rings* and *Gladiator* movies. Now, even a decade later, we often go back and watch these films again and again.

As a special gift upon completion of Aidan's rites of passage journey at the age of 13, I gave him a life-sized replica of Gandalf's white staff as a symbol of what I consider the pinnacle of manhood, the Sage. He readily accepted it with honor, and then he promptly hung it on the wall of his bedroom. It stayed there, untouched, for the next six years until he moved out of that bedroom and went to college.

For his 18th birthday, to symbolize his move out of the house and into his life as a young warrior in the world, I gave Aidan the reforged sword of Aragorn, *Anduril,* also a life-sized replica with a leather-bound hilt and Elvish carvings along the blade. Now, as you can imagine, unlike the staff, the sword is regularly taken in hand as he engages the stance and footwork of a skilled warrior. Whenever there is a battle scene on screen, the younger boy inside him comes out, and he runs to grab the sword and swing it dangerously overhead. It is even passed around amongst his college buddies as they play-fight against imaginary enemies, whether it's the rival college's football team or the orcs invading their neighborhood at 3 a.m. These young men *need* to have a sword in hand. They need to know the power of the blade as an extension of their own power within.

Who, when watching these epic films, doesn't want to be Aragorn, Maximus, William Wallace, or Harry? Most of us are drawn to the hero and find ourselves desperately wanting to join the ranks among such masculine icons. We most easily identify with the star of the story and often forget about the crucial guide who helped set him on the right path from the beginning.

I gave my son the Gandalf staff *before* the sword because I wanted him to know the power and necessity of the guide. The warrior is only a warrior for a season; the guide influences the trajectory of the story altogether. Without him, there is no story. Behind every hero is another hero, one crucial to every epic story, who is indeed the true masculine destination. I wanted Aidan to start with the end in mind, seeing the staff hanging on his wall for years. Though he would take up the proverbial sword for a long season of his life, I wanted him to know there was something more beyond it. I wanted him to have a vision for his internal Sage even before he left boyhood to become a man.

Maybe you have begun feeling the subterranean tremors in your life also. Maybe, as you look down the future corridors of your life, you see your internal Sage standing on the other side of an impending threshold. Maybe the man inside you knows the time is coming for you to put down your sword and take up your staff. If so, you have come to the right place.

―――

QUESTIONS TO CONSIDER AND DISCUSS:

- *Describe the "Gandalfs" you have known in your life. What did it feel like to be in his presence? If you did not experience this, when are moments in your life when you wished you had someone like him? What do you wish for?*
- *What was your split-rail fence? Did you have one?*
- *What tremors do you feel inside as you consider the next season of your life as a man?*
- *What do you hope to receive as you read this book?*

2

THE MASCULINE DESTINATION

As I round the corner toward 50, I am the target of an entirely new set of advertisements. The algorithms driving social media's marketing are fascinating to observe. At times, they are downright scary in their ability to anticipate my needs and questions, while at other times they border on annoying, obnoxious, and inappropriate.

Recently, my feed has oozed with products designed for 50-something men. From hair and beard dye to follicle transplant solutions. From at-home "fitness after 50" programs to aspirin regimens for heart health. From snore-reduction aids, sleep apnea solutions, and a new line of wrinkle-reducing cream for men to supportive pouch underwear designed to assist with increasingly sagging nethers. The list abounds. But while I may find some (not all!) of these products helpful, there is one that disturbs me more than any other: AARP.

Dr. Ethel Percy Andrus founded the American Association of Retired Persons in 1958 to promote her philosophy of productive aging and to advocate for health insurance for retired people. Her work was foundational to the systems our country now has in place to provide for the needs of those age 65 and older, and I am indeed grateful.[1] In fact, if you go to the AARP website, you will find a large banner photo of people like me. The tagline states: "Anyone over 50 can enjoy the benefits of AARP membership!" The models are outdoors, walking gleefully through a vineyard. Scroll down, and you find several categories of benefits, including wealth management advice, restaurant suggestions and discounts, travel packages and special tours, diet and healthy living recommendations, ideas on how to care for aging parents, and retirement planning and preparation. In essence, the message I hear is, "As a person over 50, you have now entered the land flowing with milk and honey. Very shortly, nothing will be expected of you except managing a well-planned investment fund and wielding a well-worn travel-points-earning credit card to carry you on your merry way until you die." I am sorry, AARP, but I'm not interested in becoming a member.

The notion of retirement first surfaced in 1889 after German Chancellor Otto von Bismarck declared, "Those who are disabled from work by age and invalidity have a well-grounded claim to care from the state."[2] He aimed to make room in the workforce for the country's large unemployed youth population by incentivizing the aged to leave. Subsequently, many nations around the world, including the United States, adopted such programs for those age 65 and over. President Roosevelt signed the Social Security Act into law in 1935, saying,

> We can never insure one hundred percent of the population against one hundred percent of the hazards and vicissitudes of life, but we have tried to frame a law which will give some measure of protection to the average citizen and to his family against the loss of a job and against poverty-ridden old age.[3]

And then, in 1965, two decades after World War II, the government enacted Medicare to provide for the rising costs of healthcare of those over 65.

I do believe the heart behind these governmental acts was good, kind, and meant to be protective for the vulnerable. However, the social implications are significant. As a result, retirement became the finishing line for millions of Americans of the Boomer generation, my father's generation. Pensions and retirement funds soon enhanced the compensation packages companies offered their employees, often matching tax-free retirement contributions and increasing annuity payouts commensurate with years worked. In fact, 401(k) funds did not exist before this time. As a result, the career script profited workers to stay put, work for one company for decades, and then disappear once they hit 65 years of age.

When I arrived in Ireland last week, I flew into Dublin and quickly hopped a trans-national train to the far western Atlantic coast. Halfway through the five-hour ride, one of the conductors announced over the loudspeaker, first in Gaelic and then in English, "As we approach the next station, you will notice a large celebration and a band. We are celebrating the retirement of our driver, John, after serving Irish Rail for 49 years. Join us as we say goodbye to an old friend."

Forty-nine years. That's how old I am. John has been driving Irish trains for as long as I have been alive. This thought is both unfathomable to me and, indeed, worthy of honor. As we pulled out of that station on our onward journey, I saw John listening to a small quartet while holding a piece of cake on a paper plate. I settled back into my seat and thought, "After 49 years, I hope he gets more than a piece of cake."

I grew up watching my father build a law practice with his brother. They inherited it from my grandfather and followed the Boomer career script to a T. For 40 years he fought for justice, defending our state's civil servants in times of crisis and need. The practice grew, and owing to their business competency, they acquired several state contracts for regions beyond the Denver metro area. Even now, my father regularly shares about his most challenging cases, including the case that took him to the Supreme Court of the United States. It is a career worthy of honor.

He retired at age 65, as one does, and had a few years of play as he and my mother traveled the world. They went on several cruises, enjoyed their timeshare, and upgraded their RV. The time had finally come for his mind and heart to be free from work and to enter his long-awaited senior playtime that hung for decades like a giant carrot on the career stick. And for a brief season, play they did.

Sadly, however, at age 67, my mother began to show signs of forgetfulness and confusion. She lost her ability to write, read, and find her way in the world. Anxiety and fear crept in, and slowly over the last decade, we have watched her disappear into herself. Now, at age 77, she has no ability to care for herself, and she sits day after day in an Alzheimer's fog. My father, the loyal and good man that he is, sits next to her *every single day*. The long-imagined years of retirement have been consumed by disease, and what should have been many long years of playtime after turning 65 was lost in a mere two.

BETWEEN SILENT AND BOOMING: THE GENERATION IN-BETWEEN

I am grateful for my father's hard work and financial success. His diligence in the law practice provided me with above-average privileges.[4] I always had enough, if not more than enough. I have nothing but thankfulness in my heart towards my father for the physical life he provided me.

More and more, as the Silent (born 1925-1945) and Boomer (born 1946-1964) generations played out the retirement script and younger generations assessed the costs and benefits, we began to recognize the fallout of the plan. The path of retirement resulted in two significant disappearances for men in the Silent and Boomer generations. First, while their progeny had more access to shelter, healthy food, and education than ever before, many did not have access to their father. And the father they did have was less able to find joy in the everyday moments and had less emotional bandwidth to revel in the glory of his children. Fortunately, during these crucial years of my tumultuous teens, God provided a surrogate Sage to stand with me at the split-rail fence whose presence invited Jesus to calm the wind and waves threatening to capsize my soul. The first disappearance of a man occurs when his loyalty to his future retirement plan overrides his loyalty to those who need him now in the present.

Then, upon arrival at the finish line at age 65, after the celebratory quartets and cakes are shared, the second disappearance happens when he turns his attention to his long-awaited delights. He has postponed his dreams and plans for decades, waiting for this moment to turn the key and go. The second disappearance is when he crosses his imaginary finish line and potentially vanishes from those who want and need his presence now more than ever. Once again, the man who has the potential to be a near-and-present Sage is invited by the retirement script to leave the scene.

I am purposefully being extreme, and certainly not every 65+-year-old man has followed this script or made these choices. Even for those who have (and may be reading this book), I want you to clearly hear me say—your lifetime of hard work does indeed deserve reward, and retirement is *not* an indication of poor choices or character. There are many Sages who now live the "snowbird" lifestyle, finding comfort in the warmer climates while having the time to explore new hobbies and interests. They remain engaged in life, present to their families, and on-mission with their God-given purpose and meaning. However, the script of retirement has led far too many men away from a society that desperately needs them. Indeed, being a Sage is far more than being an old guy with strong opinions that no one wants to hear. To become the Sage is to offer generative life to the world, standing next to others at the split-rail fences of their lives.

Having witnessed the Silent and Boomer generations' disappearances and felt the absence of men both *during* and *after* their working lives, an increasing number of people have begun to declare, "I will *never* retire!" Men in Generations X, Y, Z/Millennial[5] are disillusioned with the notion of retirement, and the *golden years* spell has broken. More and more, rising generations are choosing to live a more balanced lifestyle over the course of their careers and are coming to their second half with more personal awareness and emotional intelligence than any generation since the Industrial Revolution. This bodes well for the future of mankind. We must all the more pursue the second-half Sage within us with clarity and intention.

I recoil at the AARP targeting of 50-year-olds like me because behind their marketing is an agenda I believe is unbiblical, outdated, and societally detrimental. To disappear and withdraw from society at any point in life will have a significant impact. However, for men over 50, the result is catastrophic. Sages create the framework and the boundaries by which a society lives. Younger men especially need the presence of a Sage to set the tone, identify the path, and point the way. Throughout history, as we look at cultures that veered significantly off course, we find the severe lack of wise Sages in their midst.

In a recent study, African zoologists discovered a fascinating trend amongst the wild male elephant population. After several violent elephant attacks on vehicles and villages, they discovered a significant lack of older male elephants in the population, having been the primary target of poaching for their large ivory tusks. Their absence on the savannah left the younger males more likely to act aggressively and brutally. Conversely, the presence of just one older male elephant impacted the younger ones so significantly that the aggression subsided and the society returned to peace.[6] For these young elephants, the mere presence of an older male created a force field of protection and good conduct. If this is true for the animal kingdom, how much more could it be true for us?

God's great design for a man's life includes all the stages, culminating in the ultimate initiation as a Sage. The world is not designed to live without second-half men because "without elders, society perishes, socially and spiritually."[7] Whether a man is 20, 30, 40, 50 or beyond, at every stage of life, he is crucial to the world's well-being and vital in the kingdom of God, especially as a Sage. A world without Sages is a lost world. For most of us, our greatest contribution is yet to come.

THE CROWN OF SPLENDOR

Ask any group of men what they consider the core characteristics of manhood are, and they will tell you some version of the following: strong, principled, disciplined, provider, protector, determined, leader, and (possibly) tender. For most, the ideal man is rugged, muscled, successful, and hardened in battle, but soft towards those he loves. For the Christian man, he soaks in the scripture, prays regularly, takes responsibility, offers justice, and establishes peace in his domain. 1 Corinthians 16:13 is often quoted to inspire men to stand up and be strong: "Be on the alert, stand firm in the faith, *act like men*, be strong."[8] All these descriptions provide a portrait of the man most of us aspire to be, and we invest our lives in becoming that man.

However, there is more. Far more. The Bible offers an even greater vision for what manhood is and could be. To become the Gladiator-like warrior or an Aragorn-like king is not the end, but it is a stepping stone towards the ultimate purpose for men: the Elder or the Sage, terms often used interchangeably to refer to older, wiser men. As Richard Rohr says, "This is human life in its crowning, and all else has been preparation and prelude for creating such a human work of art....All you have to do is meet one such shining person and you know that he or she is surely the goal of humanity and the delight of God."[9] The full realization of our humanity is not measured by the

> The full realization of our humanity is not measured by the battles we fight, the wealth we accumulate, or the kingdoms we rule, but by the depth of soul we grow in the second half of life.

battles we fight, the wealth we accumulate, or the kingdoms we rule, but by the depth of soul we grow in the second half of life.

Consider the wisdom of King Solomon from Proverbs 16:16, 31-32:

> *How much better to get wisdom than gold,*
> *to get insight rather than silver!*
> *Gray hair is a crown of splendor;*
> *it is attained in the way of righteousness.*
> *Better a patient person than a warrior,*
> *one with self-control than one who takes a city.* [10]

Life was raw and hard in the ancient Near East. Wars and famine were common, as was illness, pestilence, and loss. Life expectancy for men in biblical times was a mere 35 to 40 years,[11] which remained so until the 19th and 20th centuries when advances in medicine and technology began to extend life significantly. By the time most men turned 20, their lives were half over, yet they had merely just begun. Indeed, even Jesus's earthly father, Joseph, fades from his story shortly after Jesus's 12th birthday.[12] For a man to live long enough for his hair to turn gray was considered a "crown of splendor." Many of the Sages of the scripture are indeed older, wiser men who provide some of the most important signposts and insights ever recorded. Sages changed the course of history.

Citizens revered Elders and sought their counsel often on a variety of matters. In the New Testament, the term "elder" became synonymous with an official role in the early church. However, across the centuries and around the world, the individuals considered Elders were quite literally older and wiser people venerated by their communities. At times, we see them administering justice (Deut. 19, 21, 22, and 25 to name a few), offering counsel (Ruth 4), and representing their people to outsiders (1 Samuel 16).[13]

Interestingly, we also see that not every older man becomes an Elder. What qualifies someone to take on this societal role? Surprisingly (or not), a very similar list of qualifications arises across time and across a wide variety of tribes and cultures: first, he must be an older member of one of the group's families (i.e. he's experienced much of life and is not an outsider); second, he must be known for his generosity and hospitality; third, he must have a high character that is representative of the ethics and morals of that society; fourth, he must have a solid foundation in that society's faith, belief structures, and history; and finally, he must able to share his thoughts coherently and convincingly.[14] To become an Elder, a man did not just have to live longer; he had to earn his seat amongst the society's wise ones.

As boys and men advanced in their societies, their sights were most often set on becoming one of the Sages. While they raised families, tended flocks, fought battles, and protected their people as men, they aimed to turn gray and sit amongst the wise, knowing that the hero *behind* the hero, the guide, was truly the coveted destination of the masculine journey.

Old men who do not become Elders merely become elderly. Because they have not embraced their generative calling and pursued the path of the Sage, they just simply grow old. Rather than living from an integrated and whole self, full of vision and hope for their second half, often they experience a greater loneliness and alienation from younger generations because they have instead become "grumpy old men." Considering themselves released from the responsibility to contribute to the world, they sink into a world of complaint and "back in my day" idealizations of the past. Elderly men who have not crossed the second-half threshold continue as first-half men until they die.

> Old men who do not become Elders merely become elderly.

Living now in the 21st century, advances in science provide us twice as long to walk this earth. As a 49-year-old, I have already surpassed the life expectancy of my distant forefathers, and I have the opportunity to extend my presence and influence on this earth far beyond what was previously possible. The question is, will we embrace the role of the Sage, or delay and deny it for as long as we can? When considering the hero's journey, Joseph Campbell once said, "In the United States, the goal is not to grow old, but to remain young."[15] Whereas the human vision once included the importance of the Elder, now our society does everything possible to stave off the advancement of years and remain as fit, young, and virile as possible. We worship youthfulness and all its implications. Growing older is met with resistance and disdain, the opposite of the Bible's "crown of glory." Billions of dollars are spent annually on fitness, health, appearance, and sexual potency to help men stay and appear young. Now, I am a full proponent of stewarding the physical bodies and mental capacities God has gifted us with for as long as possible. Elders can be old *and* fit. While we may do what we can to maintain our physical and mental strength, let us also step into our God-given roles as Sages to offer our world a strength of a different kind by pursuing our true crowns.

For many of us, we have lost our way to the most important role a man can play in this life, the Sage. Henri Nouwen says it well: "Most people in our society do not want to disturb each other with the idea of death. They want a man to die without ever having realized that death was approaching."[16] Rather than extend our years of manhood by desperately pursuing the fountain of youth, what might happen if we welcomed and embraced the second half rather than attempt to avoid it, thereby missing one of the greatest opportunities God has afforded us–to be the Sage?

As we head into Part 2, together we will explore what it means to prepare for our second half and welcome it when it comes. As Dallas Willard so wisely says, "We were built to count, as water is made to run downhill. We are placed in a specific context to count in ways no one else does. That is our destiny."[17] Wisdom begins when we become aware of our context and embrace our journey head-on.

At the end of your life, your greatest contribution to the kingdom of God will not be the wealth you have accumulated, the successes you have achieved, or the power you have acquired. Your greatest legacy will be found in the recovery of the glorious masterpiece God has written into your life and putting it on display for all to know the Master.

That, my friend, is the true measure of a man.

QUESTIONS TO CONSIDER AND DISCUSS:

- *How have you engaged with the notion of retirement? What stories have you inherited there?*
- *When you consider the "pinnacle of manhood," what characteristics, thoughts, or descriptors come to mind?*
- *How does it feel to consider the most important season of your life is still ahead?*
- *In what ways does this chapter provoke you or concern you? How do you feel resistant? Accepting?*
- *What new imaginations do you have for your years ahead?*

PART TWO
THE FIRST HALF

3
THE DIVINE MASTERPIECE

A thick green blanket covers the earth here in Ireland. Walking across a field requires significant focus and strength. As my feet sink deeply into the wet peat, the ground feels more like a foam gymnastics mat than anything solid. It bounces and absorbs and welcomes my tread with each soft and gentle step. I have often marveled at the number of houses built from stone, for as I scan the horizon I can see no evidence of rock. Passing by miles of stone walls, however, I see how the grass has overcome them with layer upon layer of vegetative covering, almost consuming the partition in one solid wave of green. The stone, I now understand, is underneath the sponge of earth.

Today I wander to the water's edge, always searching for the limits of how close I can get to the Atlantic without getting sprayed by mist or swallowed by waves. The tops of the cliffs lay covered by this green blanket, and I stoop to find an uprooted sprig from the undergrowth on which I walk. I pick it up to examine this little specimen, small and easily missed in the vast expanse of water, wave, siltstone, and shale. Crowned with a tight-knit green helmet, the six-inch dome intricately unites its thousand roots into one thick stalk designed to anchor it amongst its brothers and feed it from the humus below. It reminds me of ancient Celtic images of the "tree of life," with its canopy of leaves and its many-rooted trunk, connecting heaven and earth, man and God, its upward stretch and its downward foundation. This small piece of coastal vegetation is a masterpiece, one stanza of the green poem written on this cliff alone.

The extent of God's beauty astounds me. His work is so intricate, his purpose so deeply good. There, underneath my feet, dwell these soft and welcoming sponges of life, and I walk so quickly by them, barely aware of their existence. The glory of God is written everywhere, if only we have eyes to see.

DIVINE POETRY

Embedded throughout the scripture we find a brilliantly woven thread of God's glory written into the image of every one of his sons and daughters. Starting at the dawn of creation in Genesis 1:27, the divine image, the *imago Dei,* is uniquely emblazoned onto humanity: "So God created mankind *in His own image, in the image of God* He created them; male and female He created them."[1] Amongst all the grandeur of creation—from stars to mountains, from elephants to sea urchins, from the laws of physics to the laws of love, from the green helmeted tree-of-life miniature to the ancient oak—no one and nothing reflects the glory of God's own image except humanity. This is so important, so crucial, the author of Genesis repeats it again in Genesis 5:1-2, reminding his listeners we are made *"in the likeness of God."*[2] It is a stunning display of his divine grace and immense purpose for all humanity.

The Psalmist joins the chorus, marveling at the intricacy and intentionality with which each of God's sons and daughters are crafted and formed. He sings:

> *For you created my inmost being;*
> *you knit me together in my mother's womb.*

I praise you because I am fearfully and wonderfully made;
your works are wonderful,
I know that full well.
My frame was not hidden from you
when I was made in the secret place,
when I was woven together in the depths of the earth.
Your eyes saw my unformed body;
all the days ordained for me were written in your book
before one of them came to be.[3]

Centuries later, the Apostle Paul opens his letter to the church in Ephesus, marveling again at this great truth. He writes,

Even before he made the world, God loved us and chose us in Christ to be holy and without fault in his eyes. God decided in advance to adopt us *into his own family* by bringing us to himself through Jesus Christ. This is what he wanted to do, and *it gave him great pleasure.*[4]

Long before we walked the earth, long before we even existed, we existed as a precious thought in the mind of God, deeply known and deeply loved. The very thought of you, eons before you joined the human race, brought him great delight. You made him smile and dance and celebrate. He was excited about his handiwork, and though he knew every moment and every good or sinful deed you would ever commit, he still loved the idea of you so much, he breathed you into existence.

Paul continues exploring this thought, continuing in Ephesians 2:10: "For we are God's *masterpiece*. He has created us anew in Christ Jesus, so we can do the good things he planned for us long ago."[5] Masterpiece. You are God's masterpiece. Other Bible translations render this Greek word *poeima* as handiwork, workmanship, or work of art. Indeed, it is from this Greek root that English gets the word "poem" and "poetry." Paul literally says, "For we are the *poetry of God."* Every one of us is a divine poem, his words meticulously chosen and imbued with deep meaning, the cadence of his rhyme set to a divine beat, and a participant in the great anthology of God's most prized works of art. He crafted and created each of us to reflect the image of the Divine Artist. We all look like him. Consider the words of pastor Timothy Keller:

> Do you know what it means that you are God's workmanship? What is art? Art is beautiful, art is valuable, and art is an expression of the inner being of the maker, of the artist. Imagine what that means. You're beautiful, you're valuable, and you're an expression of the very inner being of the Artist, the divine Artist, God Himself.[6]

Written into the very fabric of our individual being is the artistry, the handiwork, the poetry of God, formed and shaped to reflect his glory to the world. As his image bearers, it is our task to reveal the inner being of the Artist to the world. Jesus himself encourages us when he says in Matthew 5:14-16,

> You are the light of the world. A town built on a hill cannot be hidden. Neither do people light a lamp and put it under a bowl. Instead they put it on its stand, and it gives light to everyone in the house. In the same way, let your light shine before others, that they may see your good deeds and *glorify your Father in heaven*.[7]

May all who see the artistry emblazoned into you more fully know the face and glory of the Father.

FIRST STORY

Original to God's design for you is the image of himself he uniquely chose to write into *your* poetry. Just as every human face and every human fingerprint is unique and different, so too the glory of God's face is uniquely infused into *your* masterpiece—you and you alone. As he carefully selected every detail of who you are and who you would become, he formed you with the intent of displaying his glory to the world. The art reflects the Artist, telling the Great Story for all to see and hear.

This is your first story, your origin story. It is the man he decided eons ago should not only exist, but more importantly reflect his character to the world today. Before you were born, you were born in the mind of God. *This* is where you began. You are older than you know. And, though you are a man like me, sharing some physical, mental, and emotional similarities, we each have a uniquely emblazoned *imago Dei* written into the poetry of our lives. Only you can live your first story, and only I can live mine. As such, we are participants in the great metanarrative of God, the story of the One told through the stories of the many.

When I ask men, "What's your story?" they typically respond with a general itinerary of demographic information. "I was born in ____. I went to ___ High School and got married in ____. I have __ kids, and for work, I ____." While this may be some of the skeletal information to frame their earthly story, it is woefully insufficient to tell me the great divine purpose and narrative of their life. Would we ask the *Mona Lisa,* "What's your story?" and settle for, "Well, I hang in the Grand Gallery of the Louvre in Paris. I am 77 cm x 53 cm and made from oil paints on a simple poplar wood panel"? No! These boring details tell us nothing about the person depicted, the intent of the artist, the story of who she is, and why the artist painted her with such a sly and mischievous expression. When we ask a masterpiece about its story, our intent is to discover its origins, its purpose, the meaning behind its subtleties, and, ultimately, to meet the Master. We want to know how it came into being and why. We want the *first story*.

As fathers who initiate our sons and invite them into manhood, it is our task to call forth the glorious poetry within them. There is no generic rite of passage, no one-size-fits-all process or ritual that magically makes a man out of a boy. There are patterns, yes, and essential elements, yes, but no cookie-cutter rite is applicable to all.

No, it requires the purposeful pursuit of the father towards the son to discover who he is, read the poetry, and reveal the masterpiece written inside his life and heart. It is this *imago Dei* that is honored and blessed and brought to bear for the world to see the glory of God revealed in this boy-becoming-man.

For all men, and especially for those who grew up unfathered or under-fathered and did not have such guidance as a boy, it is our great task as adults to rediscover, or maybe find for the first time, the first story written into our lives. This is one of a man's greatest life quests. We glorify the Father most when we live fully into the original narrative he penned for us to live. This is a tremendous undertaking, one that requires intentional pursuit, a cadre of caring brothers who join you in "reading" your story with you, and an investment of time, often years. As with all quests, this is no easy task. But, to find your first story, to discover and unveil the divine masterpiece poeted into your wonderfully and fearfully crafted existence, is a quest worthy of your life.

And, as with all quests of such great worth, it will be opposed. You see, we were born into war, an assault raging against the goodness and glory of God's face. Evil wants nothing more than to mar the face of God, to desecrate that which is holy, and to diminish his glory through the defiling of his image on earth. Evil can do nothing to God Himself, and so he turns his destructive energy towards those who look like him: his image bearers. He is cunning, relentless, particular, and brazen. As humans, we lose sight of our unique first story as we do everything we can to survive the second story–the story of our unique war.

SECOND STORY

Life has always felt like a struggle for Dwayne. For as long as he can remember, he specialized in the nuances of reading his father's face as he walked up the driveway from his car after work. The way he parked, the way he opened the door, the way he took each step as he approached the front door determined how the night would go. Dwayne's mother often busied herself in the kitchen as she made her Betty Crocker casseroles and pretended her husband was a "good man," even though Dwayne witnessed her drink several shots of vodka every evening just before 5 p.m.

The younger children learned to tell time early, knowing by the feel of the air when 4:45 p.m. rolled around. Together they darted upstairs and played quietly behind closed doors before the car door slammed shut in the driveway. Dwayne was their first line of defense, most often taking the edge off their father's rage and distracting him from his siblings. But some nights, the fire inside him burned so hot, he found them nonetheless.

Down the street lived Dwayne's friend Sam. Everyone on the block liked to go to Sam's house because his mother always had homemade chocolate chip cookies in the jar and his father did not cause trouble. They had a cross hanging by the front door, a steady reminder to all who entered of the "peace that passes all understanding" and the grace that reigned in this house. Sometimes they invited Dwayne for dinner, a welcome reprieve from his home's evening routine though he often felt guilty leaving his brother and sister defenseless at 5 p.m.

Sam did not have to contend with the kind of violence Dwayne did. He felt bad for his friend, and often, they hid in the secret treehouse they built in the gulley behind their neighborhood. On the outside, Sam's family seemed to have it all together, and indeed, there was great goodness there. However, Sam could never quite articulate the ache that lived inside him still. He needed more from his father than a pat on the head, a prayer at mealtime, and an occasional "attaboy" when he scored the goal. His father provided for them, did not hit them, and took them to church. And yet, he still was not fully there. Compared to Dwayne, Sam never felt he could complain. But deep inside, he decided he must not be worth knowing if a good man like his father still did not want to know him.

As soon as Dwayne turned 16, he left, packing a bag and moving across town to live with his girlfriend. As he walked away, down that same dreaded driveway, his father screamed, "You'll never amount to anything anyway!" To spite his dad, he got a job, finished high school, and made his way to the community college, living on couches and sometimes sleeping in his car just to stay away from the house. He felt guilty for abandoning his brother and sister though he knew he was powerless to do much anyway.

Today, 23 years later, Dwayne is 39 years old, lives thousands of miles away from his parents, and has built several million-dollar companies. He has learned how to turn his pain into productive anger, powering through hard times to make things happen though sometimes he leaves relational and emotional debris in his wake. On the outside, it would seem he has "made it," and his large bank accounts and garage full of extreme sports machines might offer some proof. But inside, he feels his soul's decay. He has survived thus far but wonders how much longer his heart will hold out. His wife wonders as well.

Sam, on the other hand, stayed close to home, buying the house down the street from his parents "just in case they need me." As expected, he graduated high school with honors and attended the small Christian liberal arts college in the neighboring town just 15 miles away. Throughout college, he dutifully made it to *every* Sunday night dinner. He met his wife as a sophomore, and they married within days of graduation.

Sam now works as a product representative for a Christian book distributor and serves as the deacon of finance at their church. He has faithfully followed the color-within-the-lines good-Christian-boy picture, which has produced a modicum of safety and predictability in his life, but at times it also feels like a black-and-white movie when something inside him knows color is possible. When the family is otherwise occupied and he finds himself with an hour to himself, he walks down to the old treehouse, now in much need of repair, and remembers when he had a friend named Dwayne.

You see, both Dwayne and Sam, as divergent as their stories may be, have lost sight of their first story. In order to survive, they each found ways to "manage," to make it through the confusion, fear, loneliness, violence, emptiness, and dismissal they regularly experienced. Neither of them could be classified as a "good boy" or "bad boy," as they each have had their moments of both. Sure, Dwayne has had a few more fist fights than Sam (who has *never* fought anyone), but both of them have struggled with secret addictions to alcohol, porn, and escapism. They both have had doubts. They both have tried to love their wives and children. They both have wondered who they are and why they are even here.

For Dwayne, the enemy came young and early, showing up in his story through the fist of his father. The masterpiece of God in him was slashed by the sharp edges of violence, and his neglectful mother marred its brilliance through her efforts to deny and cover up. He left his childhood home in tatters and shreds, his holy work of art no more than a few strips of canvas from a painting no one knew. He did his best to take the remnants of his life and make something of them, trying to prove his father's words wrong. Now, sitting across from me in my counseling office, he has no context, no frame of reference, for what glorious masterpiece might still exist should God heal the torn places inside his heart. The second story has overwritten the first, and it is all Dwayne can imagine. For him, the thought of a first story is as distant as the sun. "I survived!" he yells at me. Then, more tenderly, tearfully, and with a heaving breath, he says, "I survived."

For Sam, evil showed up with more stealth. Rather than decimate through violence, evil chose instead to deaden the brilliance of his masterpiece through the dulling tedium of boredom. The outward religious actions he learned from his parents wrote for Sam a prescription for life. Follow these patterns, say these prayers, do these good deeds, and your reward will be a life that "works." The vibrant colors of his life are too much, too dangerous, too risky, and so the enemy taught him to muffle them with broad brush strokes of gray. Though the canvas remains intact, it is covered by clouds, and all the vitality and pulsating glory found there is now shrouded. A great man has been transformed into a good man, his reduction completed by the faithful actions of a lifeless servant. To consider such first story greatness is "prideful," he says. "There's nothing great about me. I'm just...I'm just here. That's all. Just here." And so, out of fear of being too much, Sam diminishes the masterpiece, not able to fathom a design of God for him other than quiet complicity with a script not his own.

Ultimately, evil's desire is to mar the face of God, to decimate the grandeur of God's own glory. He wants to supplant the King and take the throne for himself, wiping away every flicker of light with the all-consuming vacuum of darkness. And yet, he can do no such violence to the face of God himself, so he turns his wrath towards those who most reflect the face of God, his image bearers. He turns against the Dwaynes and Sams of the world, against every one of God's glory-reflecting children. The aim of the enemy is to "steal, kill, and destroy"[8] anyone and everyone whose masterpiece reveals the Master. As I said, we were born into war.

The second story, then, is the unfolding drama of evil's particular assault against each of his sons and daughters. It is the narrative of trauma endured by children, who then brilliantly learned how to survive the attack. For all of us, regardless of the nature of the vandalism against our masterpiece, it becomes the ruling narrative, the story we believe is the most true and most powerful. We grow up to walk this earth as if the second story is our story, our only story, and we forget we were once born to a King in a royal house and of a royal bloodline.

STORYWORK

Both Dwayne and Sam are first-half men. Though they live today as adult men, they live out of their second story, the story of their survival. They do their best to manage, and by many accounts, they have succeeded as men in the world. Yes, they have their issues—their marital spats, their secret addictions, their disappointments, their pains—but at least externally, they have found a way to make it through. We are brilliant survivalists after all.

But something inside them gnaws away at the survival rope, and little by little they see it becoming increasingly threadbare and close to breaking. The closer they get to midlife, the more they wonder what this life is all about. The ache and groan for a home they have never known starts to grow, and while watching a Narnia movie with their kids, they hear the God-like character named Aslan say, "*There is a magic deeper still* which [the evil witch] did not know. Her knowledge goes back only to the dawn of Time. But if she could have looked a little further back, into the stillness and the darkness *before* Time dawned, she would have read there a different incantation."[9] As their breath catches in their throats, they begin to wonder if the deeper-still magic could apply to them also.

With this growing discontent, these men show up on my counseling couch hoping for some advice on how to get through the next 40 years. Dwayne asks how to soften the edges of his rough exterior, recognizing his method of survival is razor sharp and his wife has paid a high price to be in relationship with him all these years. Sam wonders how to be a faithful man, loyal to his wife and kids and church, when he secretly fantasizes about escaping on a motorcycle and driving to Ushuaia, Argentina, the southernmost tip of South America. They both want help with their depression and anxiety. They both ask for tips on how to not blow up their lives and how to serve God even when going to church feels so empty. And the unfortunate fact is, many counselors appease their requests with prescriptions of medication, change-your-thinking programs, and the five best self-help techniques for midlife. While this may alleviate the initial symptoms for a while, none of this will help with the *actual* ailment. On the way to becoming men, they lost touch with the truest and most important parts of themselves. They forgot their first story, and most likely, they never even knew one existed beyond an echo or an ache. As Parker Palmer tells us, "We arrive in this world with birthright gifts….We are disabused of original giftedness in the first half of our lives. Then—if we are awake, aware, and able to admit our loss—we spend the second half trying to recover and reclaim the gift we once possessed."[10] In order to move into the second half of our manhood, we must do the hard work of recovering our first story…the story of the masterpiece. This is called storywork, and it is the only pathway I know towards the full and deep healing of restoration. As the Chief Curator, God is committed to the restoration of his artwork. The gospel promises to renew all things and to bring all of creation *back* to its original design. He will not make a new world, but he will make the world new…again. Resurrection. Restoration. Renewal. Regeneration. Rebirth. These are his promises.

BURNING THE BRACKEN

The other day, on my way into the larger Irish town 20 kilometers from my cottage, I noticed plumes of smoke rising from the mountain. Mostly covered by lush green grass, large quartered-off sectors of the hillside look dull and brown, almost ragged and clearly unpassable by human or animal alike. Still without trees, these sections of land appear daunting and foreboding. I asked the bus passenger next to me about the smoke. He replied in a heavy Irish accent, "Oh, that's the farmer burning off the bracken and gorse. Every couple of years, they do that to make space for the grass. Otherwise, the thicket gets too coarse, and the land is useless. Nothing can live there. Sheep get tangled in the thorns. It's nasty stuff, so he burns it during winter. By spring, the ashes feed the grass, and the green returns where it's supposed to." I learned bracken is an invasive fern, and gorse, though starting with a short-lived yellow flower, turns its long shoots into thorny spears that intertwine to create a patch of briar so thick and dangerous that even the rabbits find shelter elsewhere.

I understand the danger of bracken and gorse. Though somewhat contained on the sides of the narrow Irish single-track roads, the far-reaching spiky tentacles reach out to attack and capture passers-by. Thus far, its thorns have torn a hole in my backpack and snagged the arm of my favorite sweatshirt. I cannot imagine the damage it would do if surrounded by these spiky razors.

But somewhere underneath all that bracken and gorse, somewhere close to the earth, grows a grass that can feed a flock. When bracken and gorse are removed, the same inhospitable hillside can support life again.

In the same way, when we remember what lies *underneath* the thickets of our second stories, those parts of our inner territory designed by God to grow green with life, goodness, and glory to God's name, we partner with him to burn back the invasive species and reclaim that which is rightfully ours. Just as the farmer tends to his land and flock, so too must we tend to the story of our hearts.

This involves hard, intentional, and guided exploration of our childhood stories, searching the ruins of our past for clues of the handiwork written into our lives. We must return to the past to regain a vision for our future, and then bring it into our present to walk out moment by moment. This work in our stories, or "storywork," is some of the most powerful and transformational work I have ever witnessed, both personally and professionally. In my opinion, it is the work of the gospel as we partner with God to restore and redeem that which he originally created within us. He wants to make us new again, healing the brokenhearted, binding up our wounds, and setting free those parts of us that have been prisoners of this dark and evil war.[11]

> **We must return to the past to regain a vision for our future, and then bring it into our present to walk out moment by moment.**

No man can do this work alone. He needs a trusted guide and a band of faithful brothers to journey with him.[12] No one can see his own face. Without a mirror, he cannot tell what he looks like. He needs others to witness his stories of harm and reflect his stories of good. He needs the God who is *with,* Emmanuel, to come alongside him and restore that which has been lost.

At the same time, no other man can do this for you. You are the only one who can recover your own heart. For the sake of your family, legacy, community, and God's kingdom, let us be men who go "deeper still" and find amongst the ashes of our lives the remnants of our masterpiece. And as we do, we will come to know the Master just a little bit more.

QUESTIONS TO CONSIDER AND DISCUSS:

- *Where do you find yourself in the stories of Dwayne and Sam? Where do you connect? Where do you not?*
- *When you consider the notion of God's divine poetry written into your life, what emerges from within you?*
- *In what ways have you learned how to survive your life, starting from the time you were a young boy?*
- *As you consider your "unique war," what words would you use to describe it to someone else?*
- *With whom can you share these stories?*

4
THE FIRST PASSAGE OF A MAN'S LIFE

Not too many years ago, I invited my then 12-year-old son into a year-long journey of becoming a man. I will never forget his wide-eyed and fearful look as he grappled with the ramifications of what I proposed. He knew I intended to test his soul and invite him into the company of men by passing through a series of mental, emotional, and physical challenges. None of his peers had experienced anything like this, yet he knew within his growing, boy-becoming-man heart this was exactly what he needed and wanted.

You see, "every male carries a deep, heart-level question: *Am I a man?* It is a haunting question that *must* be answered."[1] Every boy knows the true nature of a man is proven and tried in the courtroom of men, and ultimately, manhood is bestowed upon him by a present and loving father. Whereas boys are born into the world, men are made by other men.

As part of a 21st century Western culture, we fail miserably in the realm of male rites of passage. Generations upon generations of ancient civilizations recognized the immense value and importance of requiring boys to prove themselves as men. The masculine energy within the boy, left untempered and untended, will grow from a matchstick into a blaze, and as the wise African proverb states, "If we don't initiate our boys, they will burn down the village to feel the heat."[2]

Far too many uninitiated men walk our streets and fill our courtrooms, boardrooms, and bedrooms, attempting to answer the *"am I a man?"* question for themselves. Some pursue power, position, and prestige to quiet the inner turmoil, believing their dominance will award them the all-valuable man card. Others, like our forefather Adam who abdicated his responsibilities and stood by while evil seduced the world, choose instead to disappear into video games, parties, porn, or passivity. Either way, uninitiated men surround us.

It is with this initiatory intention I summoned my son to an experiential rite of passage, clearly marking for him the threshold between boy and man. As a boy, I had no such summons, and I spent the majority of my teens and young 20s wrestling with my identity, power, vigor, and fallout. To correct this wrong, together with a tribe of other like-minded fathers, we intended to transform the next generation of men by starting with our own family trees.[3]

Now a decade later, as a 22-year-old young man, my son's life clearly reveals the evidence of this passage. He has poise, presence, and purpose, knowing his own self well and with a certainty that surpasses his peers. He knows who he is. He remains, however, a young man, still in the early hours of his lifetime, making bold statements and naïve mistakes that only time and experience can teach. And yet, he has an inner foundation *as a man* that has been tested and blessed, and I am proud to call him my son. He has learned that being a man does not mean you always know what to do. It means knowing who you are.

As I have witnessed other fathers stepping into this space with their boys, I see similar shifts as I did with my son. It is a journey like none other, and it forever changes the trajectory of a young man's future. While not all manhood issues are resolved in the matter of a year, and we all know 12-year-old boys do not magically transform into grown men, a clear and intentional rite of passage led by the father and witnessed by other men is the necessary first threshold in every boy's life. Without it, he will wander into adulthood alone, with a blaring and unanswered question that will haunt him for decades.

Ideally, the first passage of a man's life involves his father finding the man within the boy and calling him forth. This threshold, this crossing, takes the raw material of boyhood and sees within it the masterful and poetic artistry of God. Through intentional rites, the father guides the masterpiece of a man out of the boy and brings him to the world.

In a conversation with a well-known sculptor in 1883, George Pentecost asked how he created such astounding art. The sculptor answered, "'There is a beautiful angel in that block of marble, and am I going to find it? All I have to do is to knock off the outside pieces of marble, and be very careful to not cut into the angel with my chisel.'" George then recalled, "And then [the artist] returned his intent gaze *into* the marble."[4] In the same way, a father sees within the boy the emerging man and goes about the process of freeing him from the rock and calling his art into being. While the boy's mother co-labored with God to weave and create the boy's life, it is the father's calling to co-labor with God to free the man within.

> While the boy's mother co-labored with God to weave and create the boy's life, it is the father's calling to co-labor with God to free the man within.

Unfortunately, this is a woefully rare experience for most men. It was for me. I believe the great masculine mess[5] we currently find ourselves in results directly from this lack of intentional rites of passage for boys as they become men. It is our responsibility as fathers to grow the next generation of men who know God for who he is and what role they play in his great narrative, thereby living from a foundation of strength to bring restoration to the world.

For those of us who did not experience this with our fathers, we are playing catch-up, doing a mountain of internal work through counseling, men's experiences and retreats, and storywork, to fill the gap where our fathers left us hungering for their blessing and wounded from either their violence, their absence, or both. Indeed, one of the most significant tasks of the first half of a man's life is to clearly and firmly answer the question, *"Am I a man? Do I have what it takes?"* Others of us have no idea where to even start on this soul quest, and it is for this reason Restoration Project offers resources for men at every stage of the journey.

John is one such man. Now in his mid-30s, he came to counseling for a pornography addiction, convinced of his depravity and at his wit's end with his unwanted sexual behavior. Though he had managed seasons of sobriety throughout his 10-year marriage, he found himself returning to old patterns that seemed far too familiar and far too comforting. Though he was attracted to his wife, loved being with her, and confirmed "all the plumbing worked," he found himself unable to perform sexually. They tried a variety of medical solutions, including testosterone supplements, dietary changes, and even the famous "blue" pill. Nothing seemed to help. Curiously, he had no problem being aroused by porn. He was desperate for answers, wanting to quit his addictive cycles and love the woman he married. But every time they began to move toward sexual intimacy, a switch flipped and he could not continue. The words "committed" and "sex" felt incongruent, and he did not know why. Throughout our work, we discovered a key message, a core interpretation, buried in the depths of his little boy heart, one planted there by a father who led him through a rite of passage of a different kind.

As a young boy, John's father took little interest in him. When not at work, he watched TV, tinkered in the garage, or hung out with his buddies in the backyard. As the only child, John often attempted to "be with the men," but he was regularly sent back inside to "go be with the women." He drifted from childhood into his prepubescence with barely a kind word from his dad. He lived in a masculine desert.

Right around the time he turned eleven, John found that his father suddenly wanted to spend time with him. Jumping at the chance, John quickly said "Yes!" to every invitation his father extended. About once a week for a month, they hopped in the truck and went to the hardware or auto store, changed the oil, or grabbed a hamburger from McDonald's. For John, it was the best month of his life. Though the words remained few, nothing felt better than to put his arm out the window while his dad shifted into fifth gear.

But John knew it was too good to be true. After publicly establishing the "errands with the boy" pattern for John's mother to notice, things changed rapidly, and John discovered the intent behind the charade. Though he had already been exposed to porn at a friend's house one night, John was officially introduced to sex by watching his dad capitalize on these excursions to pursue other women. In many ways, his father treated this as his rite of passage. In fact, he told him so. "It's about time you learn what it means to be a man," he said demeaningly. "You have a d**k. Time to show you how to use it."

These jaunts, where John and his father "ran errands" or "went to the game," soon became his code for a tryst with a secret lover or paid sex. It started with massage parlors, parks, and motels, but at some point, a mattress appeared in the back of the truck, covered by a piece of black plastic to hide its presence. John's father would pick up a woman, drive to any number of tree groves in the area, and have intercourse with her in the bed of the truck. John had no recourse other than to stay in the truck cab, just feet away, and to listen and observe his father's abuse and use of women. One evening, John's father told him, "Some women you love, some you just f**k. That's just what it means to be a man. And now, you're in it with me. You're a partner in crime. I saw you watching. So don't go f**king tell your mother, or she'll leave us both, and then where would you be?"

From that point onward, John did what his father taught him, careening off the cliff of promiscuity, one-night-stands, and pornography addiction. "If that's what it means to be a man, then that's what I'll be," he thought. His father laid out the path of manhood, and John followed.

Now, after a miraculous encounter with Jesus in his early 20s, as an adult Christian man in a committed monogamous relationship, John found himself stuck between two competing messages. His father modeled to him that be a man meant to use and abuse women and to allow the phallus to rule the pursuit, having sex with as many as possible. On the other hand, his spiritual mentors modeled that manhood meant remaining in a committed and loving relationship, bringing his sexual self in vulnerable submission and pursuit of not just her body, but her being as well. The cognitive dissonance proved impossible to sort out, and his life spiraled into a tailspin of addiction, depression, remorse, repentance, and confusion. He loved and honored his wife, and he genuinely considered her attractive, yet anytime he felt the swell of arousal towards her, his mind defaulted to his only sexual template: consume and abuse. This confluence proved too challenging, and his body shut down, refusing to tarnish her with his shame. "I guess subconsciously I thought it was better to use porn than to use her, so I shut down in our bed," he said. "I don't know how to be with her without pornifying her." It was only as we began to unravel these core interpretations and reimagine what God's design for men might be that John was able to name his father's failure to him and begin to bless how his little boy so desperately wanted to follow in his father's footsteps, aberrant as that man was.

Once John became aware of this deeply rooted narrative, he began to pursue his own true heart. He sought out other men to see him for who he truly was, to teach him about whole and healthy manhood, and to unlearn the lessons of his father. He also received their blessing—the blessing he never got from his father, welcoming him into the company of men.

Men like John, uninitiated, under-fathered, and left alone to find their way into manhood, are everywhere. While not all boyhood experiences are as extreme as his, the lack of intentional fathering has abandoned generations of boys to become men of their own making. They are untested, unfiltered, and unaware of the impact they have on the world around them, for good or for ill. So much of the current masculine maelstrom finds its origin in men's desperate attempts to answer for themselves, "Am I a man?" and finding themselves hijacked by anything and anyone who might proffer an answer.

The more fathers can attend to the hearts of their boys with thoughtful pursuit, intentional action, and careful guidance, the more they invite Jesus to rise to the bow of the boat to calm the storm within. While an intentional rite of passage does not provide 100% protection from developing sexual addiction, or any masculine malaise for that matter,[6] it does change the tide by offering a clear path towards authentic manhood. In Malachi 4:6, speaking of the One to come, the prophet says, "He will turn the hearts of the fathers back to their children and the hearts of the children to their fathers."[7] When a father's heart is inclined towards his child, it creates within him a hopeful vision for who he can become. The father looks at the raw marble of the boy, sees the angel within, and calls him forth.

I have written extensively about the importance of an intentional male rite of passage in *Man Maker*[8] and will leave it to you to pursue further exploration on your own. The bottom line is this: no boy should be left to his own devices, his own interpretation, or his own cunning to find his way across the threshold from boy to man. This is the role of the father,[9] and when fathers neglect this God-given responsibility, decades and lives are lost in the wake.

As fathers, it is our task to initiate our boys into men, ushering them across the first threshold of manhood via the first rite of passage of a man's life. But, as men who did not receive from our fathers this clear beckoning to our masculine selves, we must contend with the chisel ourselves. It is one of the primary undertakings of the first half.

QUESTIONS TO CONSIDER AND DISCUSS:

- *How would you characterize your journey from boyhood to manhood?*
- *In what ways did your father "show up" for you and usher you through this first passage? In what ways did he fail to show up?*
- *Where have you sought the answer to the question, "Am I a man?" How has this been answered? How does it still echo in your heart?*
- *What is God inviting you to share with other men about your story of becoming a man?*
- *For fathers of sons: As you read this chapter, what rises in you? What action would you like to take as a result?*

5
THE MAN OF THE FIRST HALF

She called me on the phone, a bold high school senior seeking answers from a current student about campus life, academic rigor, and Christian community. Rounding the corner to the end of my freshman year in college, I somehow found my way onto my campus ministry leader's "who to talk to" list, and he gave my number to this prospective student from Virginia. We talked for more than an hour, swapping stories, discovering shared interests, and making bizarre connections to family and friends. That phone call changed the course of my life. And hers.

Three years later, as mere pups in the world, Beth and I married, and we started a life together. Diving headfirst into the first half of my man-life, I scrambled for a temp job, barely making ends meet, while she finished her coursework and inner-city internship in social work. My temporary position turned full time, and I became Campbell Soup's financial analyst for the Midwest region. Over a short period of time, I ascended the ranks and was soon offered a national position at the company's headquarters—a position I would turn down to instead pursue international missions.

For the next 10 years, we soldiered forth to bring the gospel to the largest unreached nation in the world. Over the course of that decade, we pushed boundaries and opened doors–multiplying our international missions staff team from 10 to 100, launching outreach bases in three new cities, and growing to include 10 nationalities on our multi-cultural team. By age 33, now with three children and the senior member of the team, I had once again ascended the ranks of the organization and was offered a position in the regional headquarters, overseeing the work in multiple countries in that part of the world.

Although I once again turned down the position, this time it was for far different reasons. Indeed, the temptation to continue climbing the proverbial ladder was great, and something in my internal "this is how a man's life should go" script begged me to accept the offer. But despite the apparent success, I felt a growing displeasure inside my soul, a deep sadness I could not identify, as well as a growing rage that at moments burned white hot for what seemed like no reason at all. From the outside, the life I lived appeared to be 100% on point. But internally, the floor was caving in, and I didn't know what to do, where to go, or who to talk to. My strength faltered, my heart edged towards despair, and my subconscious questions remained unanswered and untended. Very quickly the battles I fought, the successful career, and my marriage and children, to which I had been faithful, were unable to calm the scared and anxious younger parts of me I knew still lived inside me. Something was horribly amiss.

FIGHTING BATTLES AND RULING DOMAINS

As with most men, I love epic stories of heroes and warriors and battles between light and darkness, good and bad. There is something deep within the heart of a man that longs to conquer evil, slay dragons, win honor, and receive the crown. For millennia and across cultures,[1] the stories that inspire the hearts of men are those with heroes and villains, life and death, mystery and magic, and light prevailing over darkness.² We do not tire of this same plot and continue to pay billions of dollars annually³ to be told different versions of the same storyline.

It is written into the human code because it is the storyline of the gospel.

Earlier this year, our family had the opportunity to visit the famous Roman Colosseum. Completed in 80 A.D., this immense structure still stands as the world's largest amphitheater, hosting centuries of gladiatorial contests, reenactments of famous battles and mythical stories, animal hunts, and public executions. The Colosseum embodies conquest. Deeply identifying with Maximus Meridius from the movie *Gladiator,* my son brought with him two small glass jars. Secretly, and in the shadow of a tucked-away column, out of sight from any tour guides or security guards, he knelt down and ritualistically took some dirt in his hands, rubbing it between his palms in the same manner as the fated hero in the film. He then collected Colosseum dirt in his two containers as a take-home reminder of the courage, defiance, and power of this epic hero. Now interviewing for aerospace engineering jobs, he rubs a bit of the dirt on his palms to channel his inner Maximus and prepare for the battle ahead, even if it is just a virtual meeting.

We all want to be heroes of our own story. We know in our masculine souls we were made to be epic, and we go about building our lives in the pursuit of heroic deeds. And indeed, this marks the calling of the first half of a man's life. Be the hero, play the warrior, become a king. There is no greater appeal to this than Theodore Roosevelt's impassioned message to the crowds in Paris on April 23, 1910:

> It is not the critic who counts; not the man who points out how the strong man stumbles, or where the doer of deeds could have done them better. The credit belongs to the man who is actually in the arena, whose face is marred by dust and sweat and blood; who strives valiantly; who errs, who comes short again and again,

because there is no effort without error and shortcoming; but who does actually strive to do the deeds; who knows great enthusiasms, the great devotions; who spends himself in a worthy cause; who at the best knows in the end the triumph of high achievement, and who at the worst, if he fails, at least fails while daring greatly, so that his place shall never be with those cold and timid souls who neither know victory nor defeat.[4]

Much could be said about the modern masculine journey. Indeed, the world needs wholehearted men to offer themselves on behalf of something greater, to lead and guide and sacrifice. Far too many men falter at the gate, choosing instead to live their lives in pursuit of selfish ambition and too-small stories. The enemy of our hearts wants to hijack our masculine power and castrate our potency, to overrun our kingdoms and take us and those in our care captive. We cannot allow this to happen. We find ourselves in the middle of a masculine crisis of wayward and lost men. As Morgan Snyder says,

> The journey to becoming the kind of wholehearted man to whom God can gladly entrust the care of his kingdom will require courage, vulnerability, and beyond all, love. To open your masculine heart to receive a love that is being made available more deeply than you might even imagine. In order to do that, you must choose whether to risk being honestly vulnerable about where you are in your story.[5]

Indeed, in the first half of our lives as men, we must make the brave choice to live from our whole heart and whole story.

This requires a courage far too many men simply cannot find within them, so they spend their lives "fooling about with drink and sex and ambition when infinite joy is

True followers of Jesus, however, do not settle for small stories.

offered us, like an ignorant child who wants to go on making mud pies in a slum because he cannot imagine what is meant by the offer of a holiday at the sea. We are far too easily pleased."[6] True followers of Jesus, however, do not settle for small stories. Instead we find our way on the journey of manhood by noting the signposts and plotting a course from boyhood to manhood. As we proceed through the stages of first-half maturity, we eventually find ourselves at the threshold of the second half.

Drawn from my own experience, study, and the wisdom of several Sages before me,[7] I identify six concentric stages of a man's life. Like rings on a maturing tree, each new stage absorbs the previous one, adding to it as it grows, yet never losing the lessons or stories held there. These include the Innocent Boy, the Phallic Man, the Zealous Warrior, the Wounded Man, the Restored King, and the Wise Sage. I briefly describe them here to help orient and invite you to consider where and how you have engaged (or not) these seasons in your own life, and therefore, what remains in your first half to further explore as you turn toward the second passage into Sage.

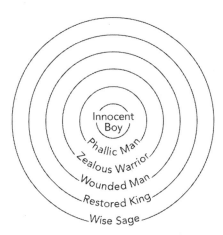

The Innocent Boy lives in the preteen season of life, where innocence and naïveté are both known and experienced. He is carefree and full of life's energy, exploring the world as a playground. At times he is sweet and tender, willing to cuddle and be cared for, and at other times he fashions spears from sticks, climbs trees, slays imaginary dragons, plays the violin, obsesses over dinosaurs, collects seashells, or learns how to throw a touchdown. And yet, at some point in this window of boyhood innocence, evil comes with its second-story graffiti and, with a vengeance, begins to mar the masterpiece within.

The Phallic Man awakens the teenage boy with his natural transition into and through puberty. He discovers his penis, and suddenly his sexual eyes open to the great world around him. He becomes aware of bodies, and as is common for middle school boys, everything involves innuendo of some kind. He experiences attraction and awareness and learns what it means to "fall in love." He also experiences the ache of aloneness and learns to pursue companionship and avoid rejection. Here, the enemy often hijacks his emotional heart by setting sexual traps designed to create experiences of false intimacy and false connection in order to keep him from ever truly knowing the intimacy of God.

The Zealous Warrior takes his hardened muscles, the physical and mental prowess he gains in his 20s and 30s, and brings them to the battlefield. With all the warrior energy, he sets out on the hero's journey, ready to conquer the hills of career, family, faith, wealth, and reputation. He presses and builds, and he digs deep to fight, protect, provide, and defend. Here, the enemy may confound his efforts, sending him into a tailspin of worthlessness, futility, and abdication. Or the enemy may instead fuel his ego and emphasize his battlefield accomplishments, giving him an insatiable appetite for more, making him a mercenary rather than a soldier. Regardless, surrounding every warrior are those injured by the battle, the most devastating of which are wounded by friendly fire.

The Wounded Man limps from the arena with injuries to body, soul, and spirit. Despite his most valiant efforts, he has left it all out on the field, and it was not enough. Somewhere in his 30s and 40s, he comes to the end of himself, and he cannot fight the battle anymore. He enters a season of profound disorientation and falls off the cliffs of depression, anxiety, lost identity, purposelessness, loss, and grief. He has a choice: to engage the suffering, to deny it, or to allow it to fester in his soul. The enemy attempts to convince him of life's pointlessness, hoping he will give up arms and instead lead a life of quiet desperation, only to die with the song still in his heart.[8] Or, afraid to enter the next stage, he returns to his Warrior, convinced his woundedness is a sign of weakness, and therefore, it should be conquered rather than engaged.

The Restored King rises from the ashes of the Wounded Man, not because he has pushed his way through or redoubled his efforts to get back to the battlefield, but instead he has come to a more centered place within himself, knowing who he is, what he is capable of, and getting increasing glimpses of his "why?" Now in his 40s and 50s, having suffered well and long, he establishes a domain and brings peace and strength to those around him. He has spent the first decades of his life finding himself, and now, he has the knowledge, influence, and ability to put it into action. The enemy, however, is near at hand, tempting him just as he tempted Jesus with more power, position, and prestige, where he is in danger of becoming either a power-hungry tyrant or falling prey to someone else's new script for his life.

All five of these stages of a man's life fall within his first half, and it is only the sixth that falls in the second. They build on one another, and rather than moving from one phase to the next in a linear multi-step process, each phase subsumes the previous ones. Similar to how we learn how to play a musical instrument, the advanced musician *absorbs* the beginner lessons and continues to utilize the skills learned early in the process as he advances in his ability. So, for example, the Warrior Man has *incorporated* the Innocent Boy and the Phallic Man into his being. The Warrior is still sexual, and he also still has a memory, distant as it may be, of what boyhood play and imagination feels like. Likewise, the Restored King has integrated the previous four stages, learning from them their valuable lessons of how to play, pursue, fight, and grieve.

Along the way, however, many men remain stuck in various stages of the masculine journey, caught in a quagmire of small stories and hijacked attention. For example, in what has been termed the "extended adolescence," many young men in their 20s and even 30s live in their parents' basement, unmotivated to work and solely focused on their video game battles (or what my friend Craig[9] calls "adventure porn"). Other countless men find themselves trapped in sexual addictions, unable to break free from the cycles of shame, objectification, and self-abuse. Still others have gotten drunk on the thrill of conquest, always looking for ways to conquer new mountains or take new territory, whether entrepreneurial ventures, political power, "lost nations" for the kingdom, or ascending levels of influence and leadership in their career. Far too many men stay kings, fearful that if they pass their position or power to another, they will lose all they have fought for, and possibly even lose themselves. As Gail Sheehy says, "But unless he also works on becoming a person beyond the person he has already mastered, he will stop growing."[10] The second half of a man's life, moving from man to Sage, can only come when he intentionally does the hard work of *becoming* the Sage. This is the threshold of the second passage, which every man must cross if he wishes to enter into the second half.

The Wise Sage emerges when a man steps beyond the story of his life, looking back over the seasons he has lived, the relationships he has had, the battles he has fought, the dark valleys and dry deserts he has traversed, and the domains he has ruled, and sees it all with a posture of curiosity, generosity, and deep contentedness. The Sage lives as a *generative* person, drawing from the abundance of his inner life that no longer needs to prove itself as dominant or superior. He has done the work in his first half to welcome home all the broken parts of himself he lost along the way. He discovers a new freedom to participate in what Thomas Merton calls the *cosmic dance,* recognizing "the world and time are the dance of the Lord."[11] Though a man's body moves linearly through time, aging with every day in the journey toward the last and final passage, which is death, his soul does not necessarily follow suit. Just as a boy's body will pass through puberty and inevitably grow into an adult, that same boy may not actually become a man. Several in my circles call these people "boys in men's bodies" or "boys who shave." In the same way boys are born, but men are made, men do not automatically become Sages with age. Sages too are made.

As we consider the journey towards Sage, something altogether different is needed. Rohr writes, "You cannot walk the second journey with first journey tools. You need a whole new tool kit."[12] To prepare for this second passage, we must recognize the resources upon which we have thus far relied and carefully and intentionally lay down our defenses, take off our armor, collect our abandoned and exiled younger parts, and step over the threshold of this next passage with clarity of mind and a sober heart.

QUESTIONS TO CONSIDER AND DISCUSS:

- *Consider each of the seasons of a man's life as listed in this chapter. For each stage, write or share a few words about your experience of it.*
- *How would you characterize yourself in each stage?*
- *In what ways do you find yourself still "stuck" in aspects of that stage?*
- *As you consider this, where do you experience shame?*
- *For any stages you sense you have not yet entered or completed, write a vision statement for yourself as you take the next intentional steps.*
- *Though far more will be explored with regard to the Wise Sage, what thoughts do you have even now about what lies ahead?*

- *Consider your father. What do you know about his story as it relates to these stages? On the diagram of the concentric circles, where would you place him? Where is he still stuck?*
- *What would you like to share with other men with regard to your own masculine journey through these seasons?*

6

FAILED PROJECTIONS

Rob called me into his office, a simple square room with a desk, a few filing cabinets, and fluorescent lights, located in an office park outside Chicago. A few months prior, I started working at Campbell's Soup Company as a temp, filling in for the front desk receptionist, working in the mail room, and making sure the copy machine worked properly. Though a recent college graduate with a bachelors *and* masters from a prestigious school, I struggled to find a job and was happy to get some work while my new wife Beth finished her degree. As comptroller of the region, Rob gave leadership to the company's financials and oversight to office operations.

Kind and cordial, Rob's presence always put me at ease. As I sat down in the only chair across from his desk, I knew something good was about to happen. I worked hard, even as a temp, to prove myself and to exceed expectations. I did not just type dictated letters and format spreadsheets. I taught myself the company's software, methods of sales, and uncovered the training gaps of their sales team. I reorganized the filing systems and created sales and spending reports that more adequately communicated the most vital information. I knew I had my foot in the door with a reputable company, and I wanted to prove myself worthy of more. And I did.

That day, Rob created a new position for me: Financial Analyst for the Midwest Region. No other regions had analysts, and he was excited to pioneer. Working alongside Rob, I would focus on maximizing the money invested in customer promotions, working with the sales team to leverage deals and increase revenue. Honored, I readily accepted even though I had not taken a math, business, or finance class *ever* in my college career.

My external world boldly and loudly answered the internal questions I had as a young man, *"Am I valuable? Do I mean something? Am I worth knowing, trusting, and loving?"* In college, academic success and my professors' praise met some of my heart's need. Getting married and experiencing the joys of committed companionship filled some of the void. Participating with a young-married small group at church, armed with increasing knowledge of systematic theology and church history, solidified my status in the church and offered some reassurance of my worthiness. And now, landing a full-time "adult" job with benefits, a travel budget, and a company Amex card decisively confirmed to my questioning heart that I was indeed a valid human and had something to offer the world.

Throughout our first half, with all the growth and adventure and battles and loves, we look *externally* for answers to deep *internal* questions. Perhaps we believe our jobs can fill the void within, letting us know who we are by what we do. Perhaps marriage will put an end to the emptiness inside our hearts, proving we are truly loved, cared for, and nurtured. Perhaps if we can get promoted to the next level of leadership or career and establish a greater sense of security with a better job or bigger bank account, our hearts will find rest.

We project these questions to the world, placing demands on people, positions, and programs never intended or equipped to answer them. As young men desperately searching for someone or something to confirm our value and solidify our identity, we cast our internal self-doubts onto our external world, desperate to find a reflection "out there" of our true selves "in here." We cry out asking, "Who or what is going to tend to my broken and lonely heart? Who will tell me who I am?" We project our internal insecurities, anxieties, and fears outward in hopes they will be cared for and quieted.

"I am important. Look how many friends I have in my contacts."

"When I save $10,000 in an emergency fund, I know I'll be okay."

"Once dad hears about this promotion, he'll finally say he's proud of me."

"At least my wife who said yes to marry me. I must not be all that bad."

"The guys will want to hang out with me more once I get the man cave dialed in."

"See, I'm a good man. Look how well my kids are doing."

"I must be really manly because we have sex four times a week."

"I must be a terrible man because we haven't had sex in months."

"I'll prove God's sacrifice for me was worth it. I'll lead people to faith."

The list goes on. We project our internal desperation, questions, and fears outward onto our external world and relationships, desperate to find answers no one and nothing can actually provide. We depend on others to calm our hearts, contain our anxieties, validate our worth, and affirm our dignity. These splintered-off parts of ourselves beg for someone or something to "tell me I'm going to be okay!"

PRO+JACERE

Projections are a basic mechanism of our internal psychological structure, where we take our unconscious anxieties and core questions and cast them onto those we deem able to provide an answer or quell our fears. The term is derived from the Latin *pro+jacere*, meaning to "throw before." As children, when we awake to the reality of this broken and fallen world and the fact we were not born in the Eden we were designed for, we project our angst and anxiety first onto our parents, hoping they will know how to soothe our anxious souls. However, as co-participants in the human exile from the Garden, our parents cannot bring the healing or relief we so desperately need. Then, as we grow up and eventually leave our parents, we "tend to project knowledge and power onto institutions, persons in authority and socialized roles....We assume that to act like the big people is to become one. Youth setting out on the first adulthood cannot know then that the big people are often children in big bodies and big roles."[1] We do not realize we are all projecting onto each other all the time.

I recently experienced this with my daughter. She is a fierce and lovely 18-year-old, studying at a great university. To say she is brilliant is an understatement, for her intellect and world-citizenry is truly top notch. However, just recently, she asked me to explain the world of financial investments to her, with specific questions about mortgages, real estate, and leveraging equity. While I am no expert in these arenas, I answered to the best of my ability and provided her a foundational understanding of the topics. However, behind her question was another question, one that had nothing to do with money or making wise choices. Her brilliant mind could have researched a more thorough answer within minutes. The deeper inquiry involved her fear of being caught off guard, not knowing what to do, or not being adequately provided for in the future. At that moment, she was not asking for basic investment information. Instead, she was projecting onto me her anxieties about the future and watching my response rather than listening to my answers. She wanted to know, "Am I smart enough to make it as an adult? Am I going to be okay?" Is this not the core of many of our heart's questions?

Grappling with the non-Edenic state of our existence is the psychological battle of the first half. Everywhere we go, everywhere we turn, in every relationship we enter or exit, we are seeking to resolve this question. We experience the ache for a world we know to be true but have never lived in, and we do everything in our power to create that world here and now. There is no return to Eden and no one on earth who can adequately show us the way.

And yet, in the years between the Innocent Boy and the Restored King, we do everything we can to build a life that will calm our anxiety and bring us closer to that elusive home.

"If I just push the limits of the next thrill, maybe I can experience a taste of Eden."

"If I muscle my way through the battlefield, take the next hill, land the next deal, win the next election, claim the next country for Christ, then maybe I can find the meaning that has evaded my grasp."

"If I can explore the depths of emotion, experience the most beautiful sunrise, or weep with tears moved by the most intimate worship, maybe I will stop feeling as homesick as I do."

"If I can sit down on my proverbial throne and bring peace and provision to all those in my care, ensuring the treasury is full and the castle walls are solid, then maybe I will know why I am here and what my life is all about."

The reality is we live as if we do not already know the answer. Nouwen writes,

> "We ignore what we already know with a deep-seated, intuitive knowledge–that no love or friendship, no intimate embrace or tender kiss, no community, commune or collective, no man or woman, will ever be able to satisfy our desire to be released from our lonely condition."[2]

Try as we might, nothing on earth can answer our heavenly questions. It is only as we recognize the failure of our projections and release our wives, children, friends, ministries, and careers from being the god of our life's meaning that we can move towards a whole heart. Nothing "out there" can calm the fears "in here." The most heart-wrenching truth of life on post-Edenic earth is that *no one is coming.* There is only one who can gather up those broken off parts of your soul and bring them into the healing presence of Jesus. You. You are the only one who can come for you.

As I have said, the first passage of manhood is to find the man within the boy and call him forth. But the second passage of manhood, the passage across the threshold into the second half, is to find the boy–the scared, anxious, tearful, rejected, lonely, desperate little younger self–within the man and bring him home to himself. We must re-collect our projections, those internal demands we have placed externally, and turn them instead towards ourselves. Hollis tells us,

> **It is only as we recognize the failure of our projections and release our wives, children, friends, ministries, and careers from being the god of our life's meaning that we can move towards a whole heart. Nothing "out there" can calm the fears "in here."**

> Life has a way of dissolving projections and one must, amid the disappointment and desolation, begin to take on the responsibility for one's own satisfaction. There is no one out there to save us, to take care of us, to heal the hurt. But there is a very fine person within, one we barely know, ready and willing to be our constant companion.[3]

No one can enter the second half until and unless he is willing to take responsibility for his own identity and meaning.

As such, our projections fail. No wife can care enough. No career can adequately fulfill us. No bank account balance can sufficiently calm our anxieties. No car, house, boat, or vacation can bring enough thrill or satisfaction. All our lives we demand the external to calm the internal. Try as we might, those broken and scared parts of us will never be made whole by anything or anyone outside of us. It is time we stop trying and instead gather up our broken places and bring them back to the one who can actually tend to them.

IKIGAI

Dan Buettner, a researcher with National Geographic, grew curious when he read a study about the people of Okinawa, a small Japanese island in the East China Sea. Though known for its coral reefs, amazing beaches, and World War II significance, the island has another significant claim to fame. The study showed that, on average, Okinawans live seven years longer than Americans and have one of the longest disability-free life spans on the planet.[4] Astounded by this information, Buettner set out to discover the secret to this fountain of youth.

While expecting to find correlations between this phenomenon and health, diet, exercise, social structures, or spiritual practices, what the researchers found was far more astounding. In essence, Okinawans have no concept of retirement. In fact, "[t]hey don't even have a word for it. Literally nothing in their language describes the concept of stopping work completely. Instead, one of the healthiest societies in the world has the word *ikigai* (pronounced like "icky guy"), which roughly translates to 'the reason you wake up in the morning.' It's the thing that drives you most."[5] Instead of retirement, Okinawans have meaning. These Japanese islanders have radically transformed their physical health and longevity by doing the hard internal work of discovering and living into their own meaning. They have purpose and a vision for who they are, *why* they are, and what they are to be about. Apparently, finding your own meaning is powerful enough to extend your life.

Philosophy students often joke that every philosopher who ever lived is merely asking the same question, "What is the meaning of life?" In some sense, it is true. As all of us spin as specks of dust on a hunk of rock orbiting a star traveling at 448,000 mph around a galaxy among millions of galaxies in an infinite universe our math can barely quantify. What truly is the meaning of our lives? This great question collides with our tremendous smallness in the scope of all creation. And yet, it is the core question of every human on earth. Rohr explains, "As the body cannot live without food, so the soul cannot live without meaning."[6] Our existence depends on the meaning we find.

As believers in Jesus, of course we derive significant meaning from his great narrative. We participate in a bigger story, the story of God's unfolding revelation throughout time, knowing what has been and what will be as shown to us in the scripture. This provides us with significant clarity, and it gives us great purpose and hope. And while this gives *us* meaning, what does it give *me* apart from *us*? We can know the great story of God for his people, but how can we come to know the great story of God for each individual image bearer? This, I believe, is our life's greatest quest.

And so we search. We look. We ask. We project from ourselves onto the world around us our desperate questions, *"Who am I? What am I? What is my meaning?"* Many of us spend our entire lives searching, only to find our projections failing over and over, and no one else can tell us the answer. To this, Frankl writes, "Ultimately, man should not ask what the meaning of life is...[he] can only answer to life by *answering for* his own life; to life he can only respond by being responsible."[7] We must take ownership of our own existential questions, our own meaning, and gather up our projections when we recognize the universe will not answer our heart-level questions. Only we can find the *ikigai* for our own lives.

THREE MEN YOU ALREADY KNOW

Every man has significant projections. Their identity, their purpose, and their meaning are derived from someone or something outside themselves. Ultimately, the projection will fail, and these men will be forced to grapple with an identity crisis the size of a volcanic explosion. It will not be pretty. Consider the stories of David, Marcus, and Stephen.

David spent hour upon hour on my counseling couch complaining about his wife. Married for 34 long and arduous years, she finally gave him an ultimatum: "Go to counseling, or I'm out." Frustrated but obedient, he showed up weekly for several months with nothing new to say. "She won't listen to my music. She won't go on vacation with me. She always does what she wants but never gives me the freedom to do what I want. She spends *my* money but complains when I buy a new car. She...She...She..." I soon discovered if I did not interrupt or direct, the entire hour could pass without him taking a single breath.

By week three I gave him some boundaries, telling him I would listen for 10 minutes about his wife and then pause him to transition to talking about himself. I even set a timer. It worked only marginally for about a third of the time. The force of this man's complaints crashed like a tidal wave, and it took all of me to not be swallowed up by the undertow. You see, David had so deeply and permanently attached his identity, purpose, and meaning to his wife and marriage he no longer had a self to talk about. It is no wonder she collapsed under the crushing weight of his projections.

Tenured university professor Marcus felt devastated by his son's choices. Following in the footsteps of his military father's methods of parenting, Marcus raised his children with clear expectations, a firm hand, and all the best Christian parenting practices, including daily devotions, weekly church and youth group, and a habit of saying "yes, sir" and "yes, ma'am" to every older adult. After his son's attempted suicide, Marcus asked him, "Why? Why would you try to kill yourself?" His son Jon answered, "Because I'm gay, and I knew you would never be okay with that." In session with me, Marcus admitted, "He's right. How could I be a loving Christian father and do all the right things and raise him in all the right ways and he *still* betrays me?" Marcus had so significantly attached his identity as a successful Christian father to Jon's life, Jon had no room to breathe. His attempt at strangling himself stood as a physical representation of his life's experience with his dad.

Rarely would Stephen return my phone calls or emails. He would contact me for a session but then disappear for weeks as I attempted to schedule a time to meet. As a top executive of one of the nation's leading streaming services, he worked nearly 100 hours a week and barely had time to drive home and back to the office the next day. Stephen now lived in New York in a luxury penthouse apartment complete with bellman, rooftop hot tub, and views of Central Park, all conciliations to his wife after moving his family four times in two-and-a-half years in pursuit of his "dream job." He originally reached out to me for counseling, having heard through a colleague that his "sharp edges were getting sharper," and he needed to "take care of that." We only met a few times, always smashed in-between two of his important calls or meetings. At one point he said, "I've been doing this job for four months now, and I'm a bit surprised I don't feel better about myself." "I'm not surprised," I replied. I never heard from him again.

These three men have mortgaged their hearts to others, desperate to find themselves in their faces. For David, it's his wife; for Marcus, his son; and for Stephen, his job and career. Each of them mines their projection for validation, exhausting their wives, children, and colleagues in their pursuit of identity and meaning. Ultimately, the projection will fail, and these men will grapple with an identity crisis the size of a volcanic explosion. It will not be pretty.

The fact is, we all know these men because we know ourselves. While we can shake our heads at the apparent foolishness we see in each of their stories, we must see the log in our own eyes first. From an early age, we project onto the world our desperate plea for someone to please tell us who we are. Only when we take responsibility for ourselves and unattach our core questions from the external, letting the world off the hook, and then reincorporate our splintered selves will we be able to move into the Sage. Projections cannot pass the second-half threshold.

I RELIEVE YOU OF YOUR DUTIES

Daniel called me in the middle of an eight-week pastoral sabbatical, a much-needed reprieve from the grind of ministry for the past seven years. During the first few weeks, he took a short vacation with his wife, and then he turned towards the mountains for some time alone in the backwoods. When he hit the midpoint of his sabbatical, he began to wonder about his relationships, particularly his 21-year marriage as well as the friendships he had with his elders, the men who planted the church with him seven years ago.

"I don't know why," he said during one of our sabbatical coaching sessions, "but I just don't feel like she gets me. I know she loves me and is committed to me. But she's just...not...filling me up or meeting me where I am. And neither are the guys. Yeah, we all have our quirks and everything, and we've come to love those annoying parts of each other. But somehow they just can't seem to care for me the way brothers should, you know?"

"I do know," I replied. "I do know how scary it can be to have close and intimate relationships like you have, and still not feel like they are meeting you where you most need it."

"Yeah, exactly," he said as he grabbed a tissue.

"What would it be like to relieve them of duty?" I gently asked.

Looking up, with both curiosity and anger in his eyes, Daniel asked, "What do you mean?"

"What if it's not their job to tell you who you are?"

"Then whose job is it?" he said with a tinge of spite.

"What if it's yours?" I wondered aloud.

"You mean, *I* am the one to tell me who I am and why I'm here?" his voice softened with the possibility.

"Yeah, I think so. What does your life tell you? What does it ask of you?"

My question opened the door for a deluge of thought, perspective, tears, worries, frustrations, and then...clarity. He talked about his passions, his calling, and the concerns that most broke his heart.

He reviewed his current role with new eyes, recognizing those parts he loved and felt alive and those parts he played because "that's just what pastors are supposed to do." By the end of our session, Daniel looked at me with a new boldness on his face. In prayerful submission, he turned to God and named his wife and each of the elders in turn, saying, "I relieve you of your duties."

In that moment, Daniel took a big step toward the second half of his life. He recognized the significance of his projections, all those questions he pinned onto others in a desperate search for answers. He went to each person in his mind and prayerfully retrieved that which was not theirs to own, but rather his responsibility. He recognized how he had unfairly demanded them to fill a void inside him that only he could fill. In those moments, Jesus gently tended to his heart, joining with him in sorrow over his unfulfilled needs and the realization that no one on earth can truly answer his pleas for healing, identity, and meaning.

To intentionally pass the threshold into the second half, we must take responsibility for our own lives, not looking externally but *internally* for the meaning we are so desperate to find. Ultimately, our projections will fail us. Our wives, jobs, children, church, community, parents, and friends will fail to provide us the meaning of our lives. We must relieve them of all of these duties and free them to be who they are, not who we need them to be for us. Angeles Arrien writes, "The second half of life presents us with the opportunity to develop increased depth, integrity, and character—or not. The choice is always ours."[8] Unless we make this hard yet necessary choice, we cannot become the Sage. We will remain stuck searching the world for an answer buried within our own soul.

QUESTIONS TO CONSIDER AND DISCUSS:

- *What questions are you projecting onto your external world (i.e. your job, ministry, marriage, children, friends, church)? What answer are you waiting for them to offer?*
- *If you were to ask your most significant relationships "what does it feel like I need from you?", what would they say? BONUS: Ask them.*
- *If you can, how would you articulate your "ikigai?" If you can't, how would you like to begin to explore and discover your meaning?*
- *Who do you need to "relieve of their duties?"*
- *What would you like to share with other men about your deepened understanding of your projections?*

The concepts of Projections and Personas (which you'll read about in the next chapter) are critical to identify and engagement as we hit midlife. However, identifying the degree to which they are present can be challenging. That's why we created the Projections & Personas Assessment so you can get a clearer sense of how these dynamics are present and may be be preventing you from moving forward. Access the free assessment here by scanning the QR code with your phone's camera.

7
PERSONAS: THE MASKS WE WEAR

Before I was born, my mother received a prophecy about me from one of her charismatic Christian friends. Spoken over me while still in the womb, the words were: "He will be a John the Baptist-type forerunner of the gospel. He will tell people about Jesus and change the world for the gospel."[1] From the moment I came into the world, I was told I had a calling and a purpose.

In addition to this spiritual banner over my life, another expectation shaped my existence, this one just as powerful though not so overtly spoken. I was born five years after my sister, who suffers from severe mental and physical disabilities. Though today she is 54 years old, she still operates at a 2-year-old level of engagement. Within the first year of my life, while not yet capable of conscious thought, I became aware of her need for me. As I learned to crawl, I taught her how to do the same. As I learned to walk, I showed her how to move her legs. As I learned how to hold a fork and play with the dogs and sit quietly when our parents needed a moment of peace, I modeled it all for her. I did not know any other life.

Whereas projections are those parts of us we put on others to fulfill a role or answer our desperate internal questions, *personas* are the masks we accept from others and wear proudly over our own faces. They are the roles we are asked to play, the people we are required to be on a stage not our own and in a script we did not write. All of us were born into an already-existing story, and we quickly adapted to the narrative and became the person those around us most needed us to be. Within minutes of my birth, I was handed two personas, one involved faith and the other involved my sister. Eager to please, little Chris strapped those masks on tight and played the part with a nuance only he could bring.

PERSONA

The word *persona* comes from the stage, where actors "put on" the person of their character as they portray them according to the author's script. It is the mask, the voice, the identity of the person represented in the unfolding drama. The persona is distinct from the actor and is for the purpose of making the audience believe the individual acting is *actually* the person they embody. In plays and on film, we say it is "well-acted" when the artist so convincingly incarnates the character's persona, the audience finds it difficult to distinguish one from the other. It is the part the actor plays.

As children, we are conscripted into a drama and required to play a part to ease the anxiety, fear, or desires of our parents. We find ways to please them and help them, even if it means staying out of their way. For some, this might involve being Mom's emotional confidante or Dad's buddy. It may mean becoming the school's top athlete in order to help Dad relive "the best years of his life." Or some children become the family's emotional lightning rod or physical punching bag, destined to contain the heat of uncontained parents. For others, they tend to the needs of their younger siblings because Mom and Dad were not ready to be parents, and they need someone else to take care of the kids. The number of roles are endless, and the masks we wear become so familiar and fused with our identities, we forget they were ever masks at all. The better we wear our masks, the more we become who the other person needs us to be. And the more "well-acted" our parts, the greater the reward we receive.

As we discussed in the last chapter, projections are the masks we put onto others, those parts of ourselves we project outward. Personas, on the other hand, are the masks we *receive* from others. We chameleon ourselves to become the person others, particularly our parents, want or need us to be. We learn how to play the part, and in the process we lose our true selves.

A boy gets his father's attention and physical affection when he throws the touchdown, and so he accepts the mask and becomes his father's second chance at quarterbacking a team.

He receives comfort when he offers comfort to his mother, who often needs a shoulder to cry on and someone who understands, solidifying his role as her counselor and confidante.

A young man is praised by his grandfather after receiving high honors at the school assembly, so he takes on the mantle of several generations' pursuit of higher and higher education.

The audience applauds loudly after his final performance of the school musical, and he finds he can hide behind the characters he plays more than the person he actually is.

The 11-year-old bully is handed a beer by his father after he beats up the kid who walked across their newly cut grass; thus, he learns to hide his fears behind the mirage of the "bad boy" and becomes more and more hardened, violent, and harsh.

Like water, we find the path of least resistance as we find our way through childhood, accepting other people's masks and wearing them with an ever-increasing sense of identity and fusion. We become who we are expected and rewarded to be. In so doing, we distance ourselves from our first story, our true masterpiece, and become something God never designed or intended.

It does not stop with childhood. From the moment we enter adult life, we are loaded with masks to portray the person we believe the world wants to see. The masculine script requires us to play certain parts, and in our desire to "play the man," we continue to accept the masks and wear them with pride.

At our first big-boy job, we put on a persona for our boss and coworkers, acting as if we know what we are doing, how things work, and how to behave. At church, we play the part of the faithful Christian man, reading our Bibles and going to the men's breakfast because that is simply what good Christian men do. For extra points, we may even go to the men's retreat or the men's accountability group to show "we are really following Christ." With our girlfriends and wives, we may have the persona of the "fun guy" or the "serious guy" or the "romantic guy," depending on what we perceive she needs and wants. While parts of our personality may be seen through the cracks of the mask, mostly we embody the man we believe will inspire her most. When we sit down with our first mortgage broker or car dealer, we put on a face that says, "I know what I'm talking about." When we are trying to get an upgrade on the airplane or get our way with a customer service representative, we put on a face we imagine will do the trick. The more these masks work, the more we transform into the mask itself. As Douglas Smith and Kenneth Murphy tell us, "Brick by brick, year by year, we build a persona—our face to the world."[2] And slowly, over the course of our first half, we become so familiar with the masks they begin to blend and morph and become more permanently affixed. Personas fill our lives in almost every way.

And the challenge is *they work*.

"I love it when you are romantic," she says after he lights the candle and serves her a home-cooked meal.

"You are such a good salesman! You're crushing it out there!" the boss says after he lands the biggest account yet.

"Men really look up to you. Thanks for being such a great spiritual leader," says the pastor at the end of a successful men's breakfast.

"Wow, you really know what you are doing with your investments. Can you teach me?" asks your brother after hearing about your portfolio at the Thanksgiving dinner table.

I am not saying your public face is entirely fake, or that nothing in your life is a genuine reflection of who you truly are. Enough of who we are leaks through and finds a way to color the masks we wear. Our personas are a mixture of truth and deception, taking who we are and bending it just enough to receive the positive reinforcement we desperately desire.

These masks are rewarded and reinforced over and over again. The more reward we receive for the faces we portray, the more solidly attached they become to our being. They fuse to our souls, and over time we lose touch with who we really are, if we ever even knew it in the first place. As a result, we settle into the personas, believing they are who we are because they represent what the world needs and wants from us. Our identity is formed by external expectation and reward rather than by internal exploration and expression. But somewhere deep within, we know "running beneath the surface of the experience I call my life, there is a deeper and truer life waiting to be acknowledged."[3] Resident in our hearts is an echo of a long-forgotten man, a memory of a not-yet-realized person living beneath the persona. Like an underground river, we can feel its roar even if we cannot see its flow. We come to the second passage of our lives when we stop long enough to wonder what lies beneath the masks we now so comfortably wear.

> We come to the second passage of our lives when we stop long enough to wonder what lies beneath the masks we now so comfortably wear.

Last week, during a ReStory™ Men's Trauma Intensive[4], a participant marveled at my ability to stay present and engaged with someone in the midst of his anger, discomfort, and grief without seeking to console or comfort him. He could not fathom *not* moving in to relieve the tension or quiet the soul. Indeed, several years ago, neither could I. You see, for years I very adeptly wore the mask of "Captain Comfort," having learned at a very young age about my family's need for peace, quiet, and calm. I mastered the art of containment and proudly mastered the skill to navigate even the most tumultuous of emotional storms. For example, when my mentally disabled sister came undone in the grocery store, forcing us to abandon the cart and retreat to the car, I played my part to quiet her down enough to stop screaming and start smiling once again. Next, I learned to console my mother, helping her regather her internal resources enough to return to the store to get groceries for the next few days. I was five years old.

The "Captain Comfort" persona remained permanently fixed to my face until, at the age of 35, a kind and gentle graduate-level counseling professor invited me to wonder what might be possible if I did not move in to dissipate the tension. As foreign as it felt, I slowly learned to give space to anger, confusion, and discomfort, allowing them to exist and, ultimately, to resolve themselves without my help. Starting in my mid-30s, I began learning how to take off the mask and show up as I am rather than as I have been expected to be. I am *still* learning. And when I can do that, new things are possible for myself and for others.

THE ECHO OF A LONG-FORGOTTEN MAN

At some point in our middle years, our homesickness catches up to us. The disparity between who we are on the outside and who we are on the inside begins to quake, sending tremors through our souls that rattle us at the core. Those men wise enough to listen find themselves returning to the Creator, wondering what unexplored territory or unexpressed handiwork may still be excavated and enlivened. Part of our midlife distress is borne from the reality that we, and our society at large, have "colluded in neglecting the whole person."[5] We have joined forces with the enemy in denying and ignoring the glory God has written into our very being.

As image bearers of God, it is our primary task to reflect his goodness and glory to the world. The art tells the story of the Artist. The poem opens a window to the heart of the Poet. The intricacy of the woodwork points to the intentionality of the Craftsman. The passage into the second half is a journey of *return* to the splendor of the Creator woven into the fabric of your being. Palmer tells us,

> We arrive in this world with birthright gifts—then we spend the first half of our lives abandoning them or letting others disabuse us of them....Then—if we are awake, aware, and able to admit our loss—we spend the second half trying to recover and reclaim the gift we once possessed.[6]

By doing so, passage into the Sage is the opportunity to bring your life back to rediscover God's masterful design.

I have had the privilege of walking with many men on the journey of their reawakening. Jacob is one such man. Slowly, Jacob raised his buried face from behind his hands, tears still forming in the corners of his big brown eyes. Moments before, he drew 17 circles on my whiteboard, giving each the name of a different mask he had come to wear. Now a 35-year-old man, at the age of 9, he was adopted in Detroit by a white family in Reno. He carried with him a worn photograph of his aunt, his last-known relative and the one who left him sitting on the steps of the downtown Catholic church. He grew up in an emotionally tense adoptive home, learning quickly how to dissipate the tension, calm his mother, and help his socially awkward father find the words to say what he needed to say. The adoptive family line had produced several electrical engineers, and though he did not share the bloodline, he followed suit and entered the same career to the immense relief of his parents and grandparents. The only person of color in his high school and church, he was regularly asked what it felt like to be so dark, so different. He worked hard to transform his accent to match the Nevadans, and now his speech was free of even the slightest hint of difference. Straight-laced and obedient, this scared boy made his way to adulthood, and now he wondered who he was and why God made him.

As he named the masks he dutifully accepted throughout his life, his face shifted and his shrunken demeanor began to open and fill the room. Slowly his back straightened, his shoulders lifted, and his crossed legs opened as he took up more room on the couch. For each role, he told one of the many stories of how he came to play that part, what the persona did to help him survive, and how he now recognized it was not truly him: straitlaced, math nerd, long-awaited son, diversity rep, white wannabe, in-a-long-line-of-engineers, typical Nevadan, uninteresting and unattractive, and so on. By the time he finished, the air shimmered with his presence and his smile could not be contained.

"Without all those masks, who are *you*, Jacob?" I asked.

"I don't know, but I'm going to find out," he replied as he vigorously erased the whiteboard.

"Do you have any inkling as to where to start?" I inquired.

Slyly, he responded, "Yes. I think it has to do with the prankster side of God."

"Oh, that sounds interesting," I said. "I can't wait to meet that guy. I have some people in my office I'll need his help with."

Over the next several months, Jacob explored the territory of his own heart. He put down the personas he had come to play, releasing them not with violence or vengeance, but with a tenderness towards his own self, knowing he *had* to play those parts in order to survive his life. Now, he followed the beacon of hope towards the discovery of himself. Nouwen tells us, "Hope prevents us from clinging to what we have and frees us to move away from the safe places and enter unknown and fearful territory."[7] It is hope and homesickness that lead us through the second passage toward a more settled and unmasked man. The long-forgotten boy who has spent the first half playing the part finally has someone to take responsibility for and tend to his broken heart. And that someone is *you*. Standing at the threshold of the second passage offers you the opportunity to recognize the man you have become may not be the man you actually are. You must leave the persona behind, as terrifying and unfamiliar as that may be, to excavate and rediscover your true self. No one can do that for you.

Nouwen continues:

> This truth is so disconcerting and painful that we are more prone to play games with our fantasies than to face the truth of our existence. Thus we keep hoping that one day we will find the man who really understands our experiences, the woman who will bring peace to our restless life, the job where we can fulfill our potentials, the book which will explain everything, and the place where we can feel at home. Such false hope leads us to make exhausting demands and prepares us for bitterness and dangerous hostility when we start discovering that nobody, and nothing, can live up to our absolutistic expectations.[8]

In the first passage from boyhood to manhood, we need a father to break us free from the confines of childhood and to offer us the blessing that deems us worthy of being considered a man among men. But for the second passage, the crossing of the threshold from man to Sage, we must take responsibility for our own lives, breaking our projections and our personas, re-collecting our internal parts, and removing our façades in order to integrate our true selves back together.

When we come to the end of ourselves, usually somewhere in our 30s and 40s as we traverse the masculine seasons between Warrior Man and Restored King, we look around and realize our projections and personas are insufficient to answer our deepest questions. The foundations upon which we have built our identities crack, and the stability we once knew dissolves into dust. For the unprepared, this opens the door for a crisis at midlife. But for the intentional few, it ushers in a season of profound awakening.

QUESTIONS TO CONSIDER AND DISCUSS:

- *If personas are the masks others have required you to wear, how would you begin to identify them?*
- *Who did you need to be for your parents? Your siblings? Your coach? Your grandparents?*
- *As an adult man now, what masks are you aware of wearing (i.e. for your church, boss, community, children)?*
- *What fears do you have with regard to removing any of these masks? Who will it upset?*
- *What would you like to share with a small group of men about the masks you have recognized in your life?*

8
MIDLIFE

I quite literally walked to the end of Europe, and there I found midlife.

When I first arrived in this remote Irish village, my host welcomed me with a thick accent and a warm smile. After orienting me to the oil heat, peat and coal fuel for the fireplace, and electricity quirks of the cottage, he proceeded to inform me of my surroundings. Having grown up in this secluded part of the country, he knew every road, house, and trail by heart. He told me the history of the pub down the street, his great-uncle's land claim after the British left in 1922, and the church's land bargain to establish a parish nearby. He pointed to the high cliffs, the steep hill, and the lowlands with a fondness born from years of living in the same small place.

Of the many directions and Gaelic names he threw at my still jet-lagged brain, one description stood out to me. As he pointed to the south, he said, "There on the top of that hill is an old World War II bunker. It's up there because that's the most westerly point of Europe. You can see everything from up there. My grandfather used to ride his bike up there every day for his watch, not looking for Nazi invaders as you might imagine, but for British ships looking to use our ports again. We would not let them because we had just gotten rid of the Brits and didn't want them back. You can actually walk up there in a few hours." And with that, a plan was hatched in my mind.

When the only sunny day in the dismal January forecast arrived, I packed a lunch and a backpack and headed to Dunmore Head. With the green glory of the Emerald Isle on full display and more sheep than I could possibly count, I arrived at the bunker a few hours later for a quick inspection. But far more intriguing to me was the edge of the world that fell off the sheer cliffs just a short hike down the other side of the hill. Very carefully, I descended the long spike of earth jutting into the sea, razor-like rocks leading the way to the end. Coming as close as I dared to the farthest point on the farthest rock, I looked down over the edge to the 100-foot drop to the water. What I saw stunned me.

There, unpassable by humans, a series of perpendicular rocks separated the waters from the north and the south. Giant swells of water rose and fell, swirled and eddied, washing over the rocks and then back again. In one moment the current rose and the very next second retreated, falling back inward onto itself with the force of its own undertow. In this space between north and south, at the far edge of Europe, I found a physical representation of what midlife feels like. Pressing and pulling, rising and falling, waters mixing from ahead and behind, neither moving forward nor backward. It is relentless in its intensity and ferocious in its power. The before and after of a man's life crashes in one place, challenging him to maintain his bearings while still holding steadfast in the midst. I sat transfixed, having walked to the end only to find the in-between of the middle.

LIFE IN THE MIDDLE

Twelve years ago we moved from Seattle to my home state of Colorado. After two decades in Chicago, Ann Arbor, the Middle East, and Seattle, it came time to move closer to family. We raised our kids with glorious but occasional visits from grandparents, aunts, uncles, and cousins, and when the moment arose for us to choose where in the United States we would like to live, we chose Colorado for a million reasons.

My parents and sister lived about an hour south, and my mother was especially thrilled about the new proximity to her grandchildren. Religiously, she drove up to spend one full day a week with our four-year-old daughter while the other kids were in school, giving my wife a much-needed break to work and manage our household of five. After about a year, however, we started noticing my mother confusing her words, bringing the same coloring book each week, and getting turned around with directions. At the time we did not realize this was the beginning of a 10-year decline into Alzheimer's. I was 38.

Suddenly, in what sociologists call the *sandwich generation*,[1] I woke up to the needs of my aging parents while still tending to the very present needs of my own young family. Just as I hit the stage of my masculine journey when I could truly lean into my passion, training, and calling, finding my footing as a counselor and ministry leader, while also getting re-established in the States after a decade overseas, I got the wind knocked out of me with my mother's diagnosis. We had moved to Colorado *for her to help*, not for them to *need help*. It felt like evil's mockery of the stride I had been so desperate to find.

Somewhere in the middle years of life, usually between ages 35 and 50, a man enters a tumult called "midlife." Like the churning waters at the end of the world, he is caught between north and south, the journey behind and the journey ahead. At times, this is incited by an experience of disruption, challenge, or loss. Perhaps his marriage or his children are struggling. Maybe he has lost a job or faced a significant financial challenge. Or, like me, a parent receives a diagnosis that changes the course of the foreseeable future. Perhaps he has come to the awareness on his own, celebrating a milestone birthday or simply by recognizing the weariness of his heart and the slow breakdown of his body.

Regardless of how he arrives, midlife is the time of a man's life when he is invited to reflect on what has been and anticipate what will yet be. The scaffolding he has built upon his projections and personas begins to wobble, and he must find something else to which he can anchor his life. While some consider this new shaky ground the beginnings of a midlife crisis, my friend Craig writes, "I call it a midlife awakening." He goes on to say, "I also notice that these questions are not just being asked by men in their 40s and 50s, but by men in their upper 20s and early 30s. This younger generation is asking questions of significance at a much earlier age than my own. That's a good thing."[2]

More and more, the existential angst a man feels as he faces who he has become on the road to where he is going arrives earlier and earlier in the masculine journey.

In an informal survey we conducted for this book, we asked men, "When does the second half of a man's life begin?" Overwhelmingly, the results showed, "When he turns 40." And while we joke about one's 40th birthday being the proverbial crest of the hill, the beginning of midlife can occur in almost any season. I have known several younger men deep in the Warrior Man season of their lives who wake up one day and feel the tumult of midlife beginning to grow. Or men in the Wounded Man stage, coming to the end of their strength and suffering significant wounds, may find they are face to face with the internal demons they buried long ago. Indeed, many men in the Restored King season regain their footing and re-emerge from their brokenness only to discover they need a new foundation on which to rebuild their lives. Even men well into their 70s and 80s, who have never truly engaged in the deeper work of the soul, may have a midlife-like experience when they must reckon with their mortality. Though commonly we call it "midlife," a more accurate description might be "the crumbling."

I consider midlife as a season rather than a moment. It is a period when a man takes stock of his life and has the opportunity to question, wonder, reimagine, and renegotiate the terms by which he is living. Midlife is the hallway, the tunnel, the passageway from the first half into the second. When a man thoughtfully and tenderly examines his life and his path thus far, he has the opportunity to wonder, as Parker Palmer did, "If I have the eyes to see—that the life I am living is not the same as the life that wants to live in me."[3] Thus far, in his decades of service to his masks and his desperate pleas for answers from his projections, what remains unlived in him begging to be seen, noticed, retrieved, and reborn?

This season offers a man an invitation to consider the script by which he is living, the stage on which he is standing, and the roles he has been conscripted to play. Palmer continues:

> Before I can tell my life what I want to do with it, I must listen to my life telling me who I am. I must listen for the truths and values at the heart of my own identity, not the standards by which I *must* live—but the standards by which I cannot help but live if I am living my own life.[4]

Midlife is the season when we evaluate our first adulthood in preparation for our second.

Many believe midlife involves grappling with questions of success, such as "What have I accomplished or not accomplished?" or "Have I met my financial, relational, leadership goals?" Others ask, "What do I have to show for myself?" or "What will be my legacy?" And while some of these questions can be the early inquiries of midlife, they cannot be the end. The deeper questions have little to do with ambition or success and far more to do with purpose, meaning, value, and identity. These questions are far more difficult to answer and require intentional and hard work to mine for answers. They are questions like, "Am I the same man on the outside as I am on the inside? Do I even know who I am on the inside? Am I living according to the masterpiece of God within me?" The man willing to engage these deeper questions will find the midlife season hard, yes, but far more clarifying and renewing than if he merely redoubled his efforts and buckled down to achieve his first-half goals.

This movement across the threshold is a metamorphosis of the soul. Just as the first passage from boy to man involves an intentional and even ritualized crossing from one essence to another, so too the transition of midlife requires a man to step over a threshold into a new life–his actual True Self. It is a reorientation of his life from the external towards the internal where he discovers who he actually is. This second passage involves "making this crucial shift from a persona-orientation to a Self-orientation. This shift is critical for the individuation process as a whole, because it is the change by which a person sheds layers of familial and cultural influence and attains some degree of uniqueness."[5] The Sage reclaims himself from all who have previously held some measure of ownership over his life. He comes to know himself, all the beautifully and wonderfully made parts of his being, and brings them to the center of his existence, maybe for the first time. He partners with God's masterful work and delights in the masterpiece enough to bring it out from the dark archives to now be put on full display. It is not a movement of pride but of dignity and worship to reclaim that which has been intricately crafted and purposefully intended to exist in the world, here, now, today.

What would the world look like if more men intentionally engaged in this midlife transition? What would the impact be on the kingdom of God if more men stepped over the second threshold awake to themselves and owning their own masterpiece?

THE MIDLIFE REFUSAL

Some call this a crisis. Indeed, to wrestle for complete ownership of your own soul is one of the most critical tasks of a man's life. It may be viewed as a crisis of identity or a crisis of purpose or meaning. However, so common is the term "midlife crisis" I often hear it used in dismissive ways, such as, "Oh, are you having a *midlife crisis!* (said with a sneer). Are you gonna go buy a new sports car or run off with your secretary?" The sad truth is far too many men come to this precipice in life and, refusing to wrestle with their internal dragons, continue to live mortgaged to an unworthy master.

Therefore, many men live their first half their entire lives, never entering the second. Yes, they may have gone through a midlife moment of sorts, when they woke up and realized something was amiss. But rather than pursue the hard internal work of the soul to recover their hearts and retrieve the lost boy within, they merely exchange their external scripts for another of the same kind. By refusing to break from their projections and personas, they remain committed to making their old script work. And so, now armed with more resources and influence than ever before in their lives, they choose to enhance the script rather than change it.

This is the man who leaves his wife for another woman, blowing up his family because he believes a new woman will make him feel more like a man. Or he buys a sports car, goes on dream vacation, or changes jobs, all for the sake of upleveling the script in hopes it will jumpstart his weary heart and bring the meaning he is so desperate to find. Another man may look over the precipice of midlife and resign himself to an unchanging life. "What else am I going to do?" he asks, believing nothing else is possible as he settles comfortably into his second-half couch. In the end, his soul becomes even more bankrupt than before, and he is left with greater debt, a broken family, and no closer to the relief he craves.

Many men ask me, "Do I have to change jobs or renovate my entire life to break free from my masks and projections?" No, internal freedom does not *require* external change. While still honoring his commitments to marriage, family, and God, the work of midlife takes him deeper into himself more than it takes him away from others. To break free does not necessitate the external of a man's life to change. He may find he can live more truthfully and wholeheartedly while continuing to deepen the work and relationships he already has. This is an internal passage, a movement of the soul to recover, or maybe discover for the first time, the masterpiece of God written into the poetry of his heart.

At the same time, when a man transforms at these levels, those who have demanded he play certain roles or wear their masks may find his midlife passage disruptive and confusing when he begins to forge his own way instead. His family and work systems may need to change with him, but when this metamorphosis happens gently, intentionally, and in love, his freedom will bring freedom for all in his world. We will explore this more deeply in Part 3.

Some men make it all the way to retirement, leaving their career persona firmly fixed on their faces, but when the retirement cake is cut and the last check is mailed, they find they have left their identity at the office door. Without a job, authority, routine, or money, they experience a catastrophic loss of self, asking, "If I don't have my work, then who am I?" I have spoken with countless men and couples who stand on the edge of this shift into retirement. They wonder, "What will it be like to have him around *all* the time?" or "Do we even love each other any more?" Even then, many of these men do not enter the second half because they have spent a lifetime crafting a retirement fantasy, awaiting the day when they can sip Mai Tais on the beach and improve their golf game. "I've worked so hard and long to get here, I might as well live it up," they say. As a result, we have golf courses full of older men still in their first half, living with their beefy persona fully intact, their sports car traded in for a matching sporty golf cart.

The common and well-known Christian version of aging involves a shift from stewarding your own resources and family to focusing more on investing your time, treasure, and talents into your community, particularly your church. As an older man, you are encouraged to "pour your life and wisdom into younger men," to disciple and mentor the next generation. Indeed, we need older men to offer themselves to younger men. However, if that older man has not done the hard work to recover his soul, his mentorship will offer mere advice based on experience and expertise rather than the soul-nurturing wisdom younger men desperately need and desire.

The offering of a truly helpful Sage is not through what he knows, but rather through his deeply seeing eyes and his thoughtfully disruptive questions that provoke and invite the younger man to chisel away at his own persona. An older man can only take a younger man as far as he himself has gone. Most of the time, young men do not want advice. If they did, they would hire an expert or consult YouTube to tell them what to do. Instead, first-half men want to know and be shown how to reclaim their lives and live out of their most authentic self. Only a true Sage can do that.

For a first-half man to prepare for and eventually engage his season of midlife, he must do the hard work of exploring his story by reviewing what he has gained from each stage of his life. He must also prepare his heart for the crucible of suffering and find those parts of his younger self he has left behind in exile, shame, or disgust. As he brings his masterpiece out of hiding and invites the young boy buried inside him to come out of the shadows and into the light, he nears the threshold of the Sage.

QUESTIONS TO CONSIDER AND DISCUSS:

- *What has been your experience of "midlife?"*
- *When rephrased as "the crumbling," what portions of your story come to mind?*

- *Consider the men in your family—your father, brothers, uncles, cousins, grandfathers, etc. What did midlife look like for them? Did they experience a "crisis"? Was there an "awakening"?*
- *When you consider midlife as the tunnel through which we travel on the passage toward Sage, where projections re-gather and personas are taken off, what work do you need to do for your own heart to prepare you for the next step?*
- *How would you like to talk about this with other men?*

9
COMING TO THE END OF OURSELVES

As a boy, I lived in the rural mountains of Colorado. Early on, I learned how to endure driving long distances, as my middle and high schools were 45 minutes away, and it took 30 minutes to get to the friend who lived closest to me. Given the often chaotic nature of my sister's needs, long before I could drive to "escape," I often took off alone into the mountain woods with nothing but my horse, two dogs, and my imagination. Adjacent to our eight acres sat a thousand-acre ranch owned by an older woman named Helen. An original homestead, the vastness of the land exceeded Helen's ability to care for it, and, other than a few roaming cattle and a herd of elk, the land remained unused and unattended. It was a gold mine for a little boy.

On long summer afternoons, I saddled up my horse and set out for an adventure. Though only 9 or 10 years old, I left for hours, merely leaving a note to inform my mother when I planned to return. Most often, the "Great Rock" called me to visit, a massive rock outcropping that dominated the surrounding landscape. To get there, I had to sneak around Helen's old cabin in what I pretended to be American Indian stealth, past the elk skeleton completely cleaned by forest creatures, and past the ancient burial grounds (I made this one up) to crest the granite skyscraper from behind. Leaving my horse at the base with an apple and a pat, I summoned the dogs to join me on the ascent, landing at the top of the moss-covered rock in time to take in the view with some homemade *pemmican*[1] as a reward.

The fierceness of the Rockies, the expansiveness of the sky, the whipping of the wind, and the nearness of the clouds filled my boy's heart with wonder and magic. I imagined the land as my vast domain and the birds and chipmunks as able to hear my commands and obey. The wind and the sky also answered to my voice, and in the magical thinking of a child, I commanded the elements to bend to my desire. I transformed from a boy into a Warrior King, and I ruled the world and everything I could see. My Innocent Boy was on full display. There, in my young mind, I joined a story much greater than my small and limited world, the chorus of worship to the Creator and became one with the rock, wind, and sky.

Not too many years later, tragedy visited my little boy's world as I watched my horse—my companion, confidante, fellow adventurer, escape vehicle, and best friend—die before my eyes. My earth-magic proved impotent to save him, and I gave up the imagination of anything magical or mystical living inside me. That glorious part of my little boy, the one who believed in realms and dreams and beyond-this-world realities, was lost, and I joined the ranks of normal, practical humans. But somewhere deep inside, I have always known there lives a mystic and a magician waiting for me to find him once more.

This inner lost boy has drawn me close with his magic a few times, especially through the fiction writing of my favorite author, Stephen Lawhead. In my mid-teens, during an especially tumultuous year of my life as an exchange student overseas, I discovered his six-volume series called the *Pendragon Cycle*. There in those pages, I found a man named Merlin, an enchanted bard and a powerful king, who ultimately resigned his kingship and committed his life to establishing the "Kingdom of Summer" by serving as chief counsel to the infamous King Arthur. Trained in the ways of a druid, bard, and Christian priest, Merlin's faith mirrored my own, giving him enough space to intimately know Jesus *and* feel creation with a closeness my boy knew and experienced often. Now, close to 40 years later, I read these books annually and consider these characters as some of my life's longest companions. And yet now, as a grown man, I find they often take a backseat, fictional characters reminiscent of a boy I left on the mountaintop long ago.

High school graduation, attending university, getting married, starting a career, launching into missions, becoming a father–all beautiful and normal experiences for a young man–led me closer and closer to the man I thought I *should* be but further away from the boy on top of that rock. As I grew up and my second story began overwriting my first, my personas fit my face like a second skin, which I happily donned for the adventure, accolades, and conformity they provided. The work I did, the teams I led, the gospel I shared, the businesses I created–all of these accomplishments testified to the beautiful grace and goodness of God, and he honored the yield of my labor in ways I could not imagine. Until I woke up one day and found myself at a crossroads, a critical decision I knew would forever alter the trajectory of the next several decades of my life.

As a 34-year-old missionary, I was offered the keys to the kingdom I previously desired to rule–an esteemed leadership position that should only be held by men 20 years my senior. I wrestled, prayed, and wrestled some more. When my opportunity finally arrived, something inside me shifted, and looking to Merlin's example, I turned away from the throne and turned towards a different path. Though I did not have words or awareness of it at the time, at age 34 I turned toward midlife and began the arduous task of slaying dragons and defeating foes of a different nature–those who claimed ownership of my life. Now, at age 49, I thank the younger man who began to wonder what happened to that little boy and set out on a quest of a different kind to find him.

I have intentionally come to the far western coast of Ireland in January, alone. The severe coastline, the angry wind and violent waves, the sheer cliffs, and the damp earth are the places I know my boy lives. I have come here for a month to write and to pursue my own heart in the process. Somewhere out there on those cliffs stands my magical little boy, orphaned and alone. There is a brilliant innocence to him, a deeply feeling earthbound core that loves the haunting echo of the cello, the shrill cry of the hawk, the bluster of the wind, and the cloud-piercing radiance of the morning sun. He has waited for decades, and so I have come.

Today, I head to the cliffs and the waves and the vastness of the sky. Today, the sun has broken through the thick clouds for but a few hours of sunlight in the shallow arc of the winter day. Today, I go to seek and to find that boy who was left so long ago.

NO MORE ROPE

At some point in the first half of a man's life, he must come to the end of himself. In all the pushing and growing, building and establishing, battling and extending, successes and failures, he wakes and finds the end of his rope. Whether he crashes into midlife like a head-on collision or slowly wakes up to the echo of a long-forgotten song, he will not enter his second half without an awareness of his limits. Rohr tells us, "Until we are led to the limits of our present game plan, and find it to be insufficient, we will not search out or find the real source, the deep well, or the constantly flowing stream."[2] For a very long and extended season, his script worked, providing him a path sufficient for the first half of his life. This is to be celebrated and honored and then left behind for deeper waters.

Several years ago, my wife and I took our children back to visit our overseas home. We left our international post and returned to the United States when our oldest was seven years old, and though we had been back separately, it had been 11 years since all of us were there together. It came time for a family trip to see their childhood home and to relive the stories surrounding their first years on the planet.

This time as tourists rather than residents, we explored the typical sites, visited the bazaars and palaces, and showed them the wonders of the ancient world. Their eyes bulged with both new appreciation and vague memories of places they had visited many times before but too long ago to fully remember. We also took them to our neighborhood, showing them the small corner market where we shopped, the boat docks where we caught the ferry, and the every-day places we frequented. We took them to the hospital and street corner where trauma came far too close, and we told them the stories of our harrowing adventures and worst tragedies.

At the end of the trip, as the sun set on our last evening, our son turned to my wife and said, "Wow, Mom. You were a real badass!" Beth smiled and glowed, and in response, she said, "Yes. Yes, I was."

While our intent was to reintroduce our children to their origin stories, the subtext of the trip involved Beth and I blessing our younger selves. We saw on those streets the young principled missionaries, working so hard to survive in a foreign world. We saw them struggling to learn the language, make friends, find community, and stay safe. We sat with them on the buses, minibuses, ferries, trams, and trains as they spent hours traversing the megacity to spend a few hours on a college campus in hopes of sharing the gospel with a few students. We joined them in the small electrician's shop down the street from their apartment as they watched on television the horrors of the 9/11 attacks. We sat with them on the benches at the park while their young children played on the playground and the other parents kept their distance from the "foreigners."

We looked back through the tunnel of time to the young man and young woman who pressed so hard to do what was right for the sake of the gospel. We honored them for their valiance and blessed them for their good hearts. We said "thank you" to them for all they did and wept with them for all they lost. Those were the most formative years of our first half. They were also some of the hardest and darkest.

When we boarded the plane to return home after that trip, something inside me settled. I took a deep breath as I watched the city disappear beneath the clouds, and I said one last thank you and then a goodbye to the younger me who lived there, fought there, and gave his life to the people of that country. He had done well, and I blessed him for it.

I also blessed him for recognizing the end of his rope. He knew he could not, *should* not, continue, and he did what he could to investigate his heart to find the life still longing to live within him. Though he received offers for promotions and exciting opportunities to continue leading the ministry in the country and region, that 34-year-old man knew he had come to the end of himself, and he instead needed to tend to the shaky inner parts of his soul. He had already tied many knots in the rope, desperate to hold on just a little longer, but eventually he found the end. I am so glad he did.

No man can enter the second half of his life until he is finished with the first. As long as he hangs on to the structures, promises, power, and drive of the first half of his life, he will not be able to engage the downward calling of the second. Rohr writes, "None of us can know much about second-half-of-life spirituality as long as we are still trying to create the family, the parenting, the security, the order, the pride that we were not given in the first half."[3]

We must bless those younger men, honor their valor, and weep with them over their losses, and then release them to the next season of their lives. They cannot enter the second half if they are still trying to make the first half work.

At the end of World War II, thousands of honor-bound Japanese soldiers came home in shame. They pledged their lives to win the Emperor's battles, and instead, they returned demoralized and defeated as Japan surrendered after the devasting bombs dropped on Hiroshima and Nagasaki in 1945. These disgraced men could not face their families or reintegrate into normal life, knowing they failed in the role as the *loyal soldier*.

Wisely, several community leaders created formalized rituals by which they publicly thanked the soldiers for their courageous service, blessed their efforts as sufficient and enough, reminded them the war was indeed over, and then discharged the loyal soldier and welcomed back the man. In so doing, they released these men from their first-half duties and returned them to society as more than soldiers.[4]

As we come to the midlife season of our lives, we must discharge our own loyal soldiers, releasing them and turning our eyes forward to what is next. Just as the Japanese soldiers needed to be ceremonially freed from their duties, so too your "loyal soldier cannot get you to the second half of life. He does not even understand it. He has not been there. He can help you 'get through hell,'...but then you have to say goodbye."[5]

The loyal soldier has served you well and has likely saved you from a host of terrors, addictions, and bad decisions. He has protected you through life's many battles, but he cannot come with you into the second half. Though his voice has been loud, faithful, and helpful, he must now be released if you are to hear the voice of God.

THE SOUL'S JOURNEY

The primary task of the first half is to develop enough ego strength to "leave father and mother,"[6] to emancipate from the childhood home and enter the world as a man. After the first passage from boy to man, he is to explore and engage the various seasons of life and learn from each the necessary lessons they have to teach. Along the way, his masculine soul grows and develops, he increases his awareness of self and others, and he becomes more "man" along the way.

At least, he's supposed to.

Many men dive headfirst into the next season of life without adequately reflecting on or incorporating the wisdom of the previous season. They move forward with increased opportunities, dominance, and influence but remain unaware of the vital growth God has intended for them along the way. Rather than becoming more "man," they remain unfinished boys in men's bodies with the power to do significant harm to themselves and those around them.

Throughout the first half, we are to read our narrative and learn as much as we can about how we are built and what we are made of. We are to discover as fully as possible the masterpiece that lives within us. But we cannot pass through the gateway of the second half to find our soul's content unless we have first attended to building the container in which it was meant to be held.

I often lead men through an exercise I call a "Full Life Review." To start, I instruct them to create a timeline of their lives, from birth through the present, and plot their significant moments. Above the line belong the positive moments—the more significant the moment, the higher above the line they are plotted. Negative or harmful moments belong below the line, with the more devastating ones further down. Together, we look at the overall story as it has unfolded over time and wonder what narrative God has been telling.[7] If needed, we stop and attend more deeply to the significantly tragic stories, where wounds of the man's heart remain open and bleeding. This is the beginning of the storywork mentioned previously.

After a man has done significant work around the traumas and tragedies of his life, recognizing the patterns he developed as a result, the survival skills he learned, and the interpretations he came to believe about himself, God, and others, he must then take the next step. He must reflect on each stage of the masculine journey and ask himself these five questions:

1) What did I learn?
2) Where did I succeed?
3) Where did I fail?

4) How am I still stuck here?
5) What part of my heart remains orphaned here?

As he spends prayerful time reflecting on these questions, he sorts through the chaff and ashes to find the treasures God has buried there. If we are to grow into our Sage with more awareness of our narrative, then we must review it with care and make notes in our own margins of what we have gained, lost, learned, forgotten, or abandoned.

STUCK

Thomas stood proudly as "king of the hill," having started and led his small biotech business from nothing to a $100M company in less than seven years. His savvy intellect and winsome personality landed him some of the most coveted government contracts, and his hiring department could not keep up with the burgeoning need for talent. Thomas's muscles accentuate his many tattoos, and his chiseled features communicate power, decisiveness, and authority. He is a force to be reckoned with in business and in life.

His wife sent him to see me, and out of deference to the only person in the world who could tell him what to do, he obliged. She had grown concerned about his occasional flashes of anger and wanted him to get "checked out."

"Well, doc, what do you want to know?" he asked after blustering into my counseling office, sitting in my chair, and leaving the couch for me.

"That's a great question," I responded. "Let's start with why you took my chair."

"Oh, gosh," he said with a false fluster in his voice. "I'm so sorry. I didn't know. Did you want to switch?"

"Not yet, but thanks for asking. I'd love to wonder with you why you immediately sat in what is obviously the therapist's chair. What's it like over there?" I inquired playfully.

"It's good. Yeah. Comfy," he responded as he bounced a few times and patted the arms of the chair with his hands.

With a slight grin, I asked, "Besides the chair's construction, what makes it comfy for you?"

"It's kinda like I belong here, you know?" he replied.

"Yes," I said, "I'm aware that is how it feels for you." I paused for a few seconds in order for my next words to have space to hang in the air between us. "Why do you belong there?"

"It's where the power is. I can see the door, the clock, out the window, and you. It's the best seat in the room," he answered, looking around as if scoping it out.

Again, I waited a few seconds to respond, taking a deep breath, intentionally slowing the pace of our engagement. "I imagine something in you is drawn to the seat of power. Am I right?" I asked.

"All the time," he nervously laughed as he started to grip the seat. I could tell my question made him uncomfortable, and he was uncomfortable with being uncomfortable, especially with another man.

After a breath, I asked, "And Thomas...what would it feel like for you to sit over here, *not* in the seat of power?" I asked as I pointed to the couch.

"I don't know. I've never sat there before," he admitted. His grip on the chair turned his knuckles white, and I could see a small patch of redness forming at the base of his throat.

I suggested, "Well, take a moment. What do you imagine it being like?"

"Powerless, off, distant, cold, alone, scary," he offered. He had both fear and hatred in his voice. Some words were said with contempt while other words sounded young.

"Those could certainly be true," I responded, "but there are other options too."

Flustered, he said, "I can't imagine. Like what?" The red spot spread further up his neck.

"Safe, relieving, peaceful, cared-for, at ease," I offered as I leaned back on the couch and spread my arms along the back. "What do you know of these feelings?"

"To be honest, nothing. I don't know what you are talking about," he confessed, laughing and pretending to be stumped. I did not buy it.

"I understand you are here because your wife wanted you to look into your flashes of anger. Is that right?" I asked matter-of-factly.

Thomas responded, "Yep. She says I'm leaking. It's not like I'm exploding or anything, just leaking. That's the word she used."

"Okay. Good to know. So next time, how about you try sitting here? I get my seat, and you get the couch where my clients sit, and I get to care for you. How does that sound?" I asked, knowing what was about to happen. The bear had officially been poked.

"Who the hell do you think you are?" he boomed. "I'm not here to talk about chairs and couches. I'm here to talk about anger!"

"Isn't that what we are talking about?" I asked compassionately, noticing out loud how his posture had just shifted–sitting up in the chair, leaning forward with his hands on his knees, looking as if he was preparing to pounce. "You just muscled up. And I only asked what it might be like for you to be cared for by someone else. That seems threatening."

"Damn right it is," he said stiffly, yet intentionally sitting back in the chair again.

"Power is a very addictive drug," I noted with as much compassion and care as I could communicate through my eyes. "Power known too young in our lives is terrifying." Again, I sat back on the couch and invited him to lean back in the chair. Together, we took a few deep breaths, and the bear turned into a cub.

Thomas responded, this time with his eyes looking at the floor, "It's all I know. It's all I've been allowed to know."

"I'm so sad to hear that, Thomas. There is more to know, Thomas," I offered. "What do you think? Are you in?"

"I'm in," he said simply, looking more like a man than the business beast he previously embodied.

Over the next several weeks, from the couch, Thomas shared how he had come from a destitute family, often with nothing but a single can of beans in the cupboard and a week to go before the next paycheck. He told me how he put himself through college, surfing couches and eating little more than ramen and food his friends could smuggle out of the dining hall. Against all odds, he graduated at the top of his class and won a prestigious internship at one of the nation's top biotech companies. After only one year, he left and launched his own company, and within the first year, Thomas made his first million. He worked out at 4 a.m. and got to the office by 5:30 a.m., crushing his daily goals by the time everyone else came in at 8 a.m. He loved the thrill of the conquest, always steam-rolling his way through his meetings and leaving his colleagues and competitors wondering what just happened.

Thomas's hunger for more became his addiction, and he became his power's mercenary. To not have the seat of power meant losing the game, and he refused to lose. He was firmly stuck in his Warrior Man and could not break free. To relinquish the power of the warrior meant leaving the safety and provision he found there, rendering him vulnerable once again. But slowly, after having another older, gentler man sit him on the couch and not attempt to take anything *from* him but instead give *to* him, his fists started to lower and he began to recognize how scared he was to fail. The flashes of anger, we discovered, were actually flashes of fear.

After some incredible work in his life and story, Thomas retrieved his heart from the mercenary and began to listen to his fear. He slowly learned from his Warrior Man the lessons of war *and* peace and allowed his heart to feel the pangs of grief.

In the same way, Caleb returned to his Wounded Man, who went bankrupt in a new startup venture, thanked him for his bold and brave efforts, and released him from thoughts of worthlessness and defeat. Patrick recovered his heart from his Phallic Man in his early 20s, listing all of the women he objectified and used as a pleasurable escape from his own life. James acknowledged his resentment and resignation as a Wounded Man, having been swallowed up in grief at the death of his mother and father in a car accident. Robert turned back towards the elders who fired him from the church he planted as a King, recognizing how his petulance cast a dark shadow over the ministry and prevented the vision from being realized.

Each of these men, after reviewing their lives one season at a time and asking incredibly brave and hard questions, found new freedom and awareness they never imagined remained buried in those fields. They intentionally *appropriated* and *absorbed* the wisdom from those seasons of their lives, mining their experience for undiscovered treasure. These men realized they could not move into the second half of their lives without completing God's intentions for the first.

TAKING RESPONSIBILITY

In the first half of a man's life, a man lives a script and a story that are mostly given to him. To survive the world in which he finds himself and the unfolding narratives that demand more of him than he has to offer, he crafts acceptable personas and wears script-ready masks. He projects his desperations, his wants, his fears, and his desires onto the world around him, asking his wife, career, children, church, and bank account to tell him who he is, what he's made of, and why he is here. Somewhere in midlife, he comes to the halting realization that no one "out there" can answer these questions for him, and he is left by himself to grapple with the realization that he is, indeed, alone.

It is in this middle ground, this space at midlife where he finds himself on the precipice of the second half, that he has a choice to make. He must "become conscious, accept responsibility for the rest of the pages and risk the largeness of life to which we are summoned."[8] It is only when he takes ownership of his journey and makes conscious those areas of his life that have remained sequestered to the subconscious that he will be able to grapple with the fact that no one is coming for him.

None of us was born in Eden. All of us have been cast out of the garden, and we now wander this earth in search of our true home. Something in our psyche knows we do not belong here but were made for another place, another kingdom. As C.S. Lewis says, "If I find in myself desires which nothing in this world can satisfy, the only logical explanation is that I was made for another world."[9] And yet, it is in *this* world we find ourselves and must grapple with the reality of how separate and alone we actually are.

"But I am not an orphan," you might say. "My parents are still alive, still married, and I had a good childhood." I am grateful when I hear comments such as this and pleased to know some families have had some approximation of what life closer to heaven might be like. *And*...all of us, including our good, kind, and present parents, were not born inside the Garden's perfection, where sin, death, darkness, and tears do not exist. They too, in all their goodness, could not return past the flaming swords of human exile but did their best to raise us outside of Eden. Yet we know, perfection does not exist anywhere but there. As a result, we all grapple with the consequences of our exile, groaning and longing for the restoration of all things and our ultimate return home.

Until then, we survive. In the first half of a man's life, he wrestles with the curse, doing everything he can to beat futility, stave off death, and find a place for his orphaned boy to belong. But someday he comes to the place in his life, whether that is at age 30 or 80 or somewhere in between, when he realizes his life actually begins twice: "The day we are born and the day we accept the radical existential fact that our life, for all its delimiting factors, is essentially ours to choose."[10]

> Every man must wake up and say to himself, "I am the only one who can take responsibility for my life. Ultimately, I am accountable. I have to deal with this."

Every man must wake up and say to himself, "I am the only one who can take responsibility for my life. Ultimately, I am accountable. I have to deal with this."

To make this move of responsibility, he must first recognize all the places where he has projected himself on to others. He identifies how significantly he has demanded his wife to certify his worthiness, his sexiness, and his validity as a man. He must reclaim from her his subconsciously dissociated self, relieving her of the blame she has carried for failing him all these years. He relieves her of the responsibility to care for his orphaned boy, requiring her to keep him safe, tend to his needs, and give him a place to belong. He individuates himself more fully, allowing her to be *her* and him to be *him*, devoid of the fear that without her, he will dissolve. He commits himself more deeply to her, coming awake to their mutual orphanhood, and offers a more generous kindness when she fails, is scared, or loses her way.

He reconsiders the demands he has placed on his children, freeing them of the responsibility of living the life he wishes he had lived. He frees them to be their own uniquely designed image bearers, to write their own stories for their own time, and gives them over to the Father who cares more deeply for them than he ever could. He turns his face of delight towards them, to all their glories and failures, and grows a spaciousness inside himself to welcome them back whenever they need refuge.

He pays off the mortgage of his identity, accepting the limited extent to which his job or career can provide meaning and purpose to his existence. He takes a deep breath when considering his successes and failures and acknowledges both as part of his journey of growth and maturity. He reclaims his right to exist as a divinely poeted son of God and detaches his identity from his ability to wrestle futility to the ground. Something deep within him settles as he comes to understand the meaning of contentment and learns to speak over himself the word "enough."

In all these areas, he takes responsibility for his own self, his True

Self. He wakes up to an awareness that "life is a matter of becoming fully and consciously who we already are, but it is a self that we largely do not know."[11] He admits no one can know him if he does not know himself and commits to the ongoing quest of discovery. There is no "arrival," but a path towards becoming more and more the man God originally designed him to be. Maturity is not a destination but a journey, and the second-half man grows in his consciousness moment by moment, becoming increasingly aware of his unconscious patterns and influences. We will never fully know the mystery and mind of God, but we are called to live as consciously as we can.

And amid this, he does not disengage from his life or commitments, pulling out and disappearing from marriage, work, children, and community. However, his posture towards these things changes as he unhitches his identity from them and turns instead to pursue the orphan boy inside. Hollis tells us, "Yet even while the outer world continues to require our efforts, we must take the turn within in order to grow, to change, to find that person who is the goal of the journey."[12] The second-half man shifts his focus from the first-half script to one much more worthy of his life—the script he co-authors with God as he discovers more and more of the masterpiece within.

MERE PREPARATION

When we come to the end of our rope, discharge the loyal soldier, and review, learn, and recover those parts of our lives left behind in our masculine journey, we are free to make the journey downward into the second half. Now unencumbered, the emerging Sage within us discovers for himself a new home, a new refuge. "The true faith journey begins at this point," Rohr tells us. "Up to now everything is mere preparation. Finally, we have a container strong enough to hold the contents of our real life."[13] The true weight, the true richness of who we are, cannot be held in first-half containers. As Jesus tells us in Mark 2:22, "And no one pours new wine into old wineskins.

Otherwise, the wine will burst the skins, and both the wine and the wineskins will be ruined. No, they pour new wine into new wineskins."[14] Just as the first passage changes the boy into a man, the second passage transforms the man yet again.

Approaching the threshold of the second half, like any significant change in our lives, can feel daunting, overwhelming, and as though we are never quite ready. Often, the closer we get, the more fierce the experience becomes. As John O'Donohue writes,

> It is a lovely testimony to the fullness and integrity of an experience or a stage of life that it intensifies toward the end into a real frontier that cannot be crossed without the heart being passionately engaged and woken up. At this threshold a great complexity of emotion comes alive: confusion, fear, excitement, sadness, hope. This is one of the reasons such vital crossings were always clothed in ritual.[15]

Moving with intention toward this passage, with an awareness of what has come before combined with a new and deep settledness about what lies ahead, prepares a man to take his first steps into the increased internal territory of the Sage.

Here on the rugged Irish coast, alone on this month-long hermitage with only sheep, a few pub patrons, and myself for company, I have stared long into the burning embers of the fire in silent and prayerful reflection over the many long, brutal, glorious, painful, and precious seasons of my life. I know God has far more for me in the years ahead as I more fully enter this season of my second half, yet I have begun to explore the forgotten landscapes of my heart and revisit some of the long-forsaken places of my soul. Not every man can briefly escape the world as I have here, yet I know every man is called to take heed of the changing seasons of his life and mark them with purpose and intention. O'Donohue continues,

It is wise in your own life to be able to recognize and acknowledge the key thresholds: to take your time; to feel all the varieties of presence that accrue there; to listen inward with complete attention until you hear the inner voice calling you forward. The time has come to cross.[16]

You will know when it is time. And when it is, cross.

QUESTIONS TO CONSIDER AND DISCUSS:

- *Consider the five questions presented in the "Full Life Review." Spend some time reflecting on each season of your life thus far, and wonder what treasure might be buried there:*

What did you learn?
Where did you succeed?
Where did you fail?
How are you still stuck here?
What part of your heart remains orphaned here?

- *Who do you believe is responsible to come for you? Who do you need to release?*
- *How would you like to bless your younger man, honoring him for his efforts, valor, vision, survival, and hope, and then release him to move onward in his journey?*

PART THREE
THE SAGE OF THE SECOND HALF

As I have already mentioned, I am on the front end of this journey. I stand just across the threshold, still able to see through the passageway to the journey behind but holding a vision and a hope for what is yet to come. I agree with Rilke when he says, "And then the knowledge comes to me that I have space within me for a second, timeless, larger life."[1] Yes, there is room now within me for yet another larger life. While I cannot yet completely describe what it feels like to be a fully developed Sage, I do know what it feels like to be *with* one. And, like many of us, I also know how it feels to be in the presence of a man who *should* be a Sage but has not yet taken those vital steps.

When I consider the Sages I have had the privilege of knowing, as well as take a broad review of the writings and teachings of venerated Sages about the second half of life, six repeated themes emerge regarding the hallmark characteristics of such men. If indeed, "the second half of life is the ultimate initiation,"[2] those of us on the journey through this rite of passage need to orient ourselves to the road ahead. Though each man's journey is as unique as the masterpiece written into his heart by God, I find it helpful to explore the qualities of the man I am seeking to become.

The six distinctive aspects that mark the presence of a Sage are: (1) settled contentment; (2) spacious inner hospitality; (3) generous spirituality; (4) patient suffering; (5) welcome solitude; and (6) True Self integration. Together, let us explore each of these hallmarks, recognizing the journey of the second-half Sage is a lifelong path. Slowly, as we enter and further explore this new Sage territory, like the characters in *The Chronicles of Narnia* upon arriving in the new Narnia, I hope we will exclaim, "I have come home at last! This is my real country! I belong here. This is the land I have been looking for all my life, though I never knew it till now...Come further up, come further in!"[3]

Let us explore what it means to be a Sage.

10

THE SAGE'S ENOUGH: SETTLED CONTENTMENT

It is a very simple life here in Dhún Chaoin, Ireland. The homes are mostly single-story cottages sitting on small plots of land. Despite the damp weather, clotheslines hold the week's laundry, and smoke rising from the chimney is the only indicator someone is home. Each day, residents emerge to do basic chores, sometimes stroll through the single-lane roads on their way to nowhere, or simply enjoy the brisk air and the vast green hills surrounding this sleepy village. The men meet up at the pub for a pint or two as the sun sets around 4 o'clock on January afternoons. There is an air of contentment in this place, and it is seeping into my soul.

It reminds me often of the Apostle Paul. Any student of the scripture knows the tumultuous life he lived, the many challenges he faced, and the significant suffering he endured. We first meet him as a young man named Saul in Acts 7, determined to destroy the church, killing and imprisoning Christians as he fully embraces the Zealous Warrior stage of his life. As a devout Jew following the Hebraic law to the letter, he owns a mission at the stoning of Stephen: to wage war on those who follow the man named Jesus.

Though feared for his vehemence throughout the region, Saul has a jolting encounter with Jesus in Acts 9, transforming him into one of our great spiritual fathers. Now reborn as Paul, throughout the remainder of Acts and the bulk of the New Testament, we witness this man's tumultuous journey. He lives a hard life, suffers much, and turns all of his Zealous Warrior energy toward sanctifying the church instead of killing her.

But somewhere on his journey of manhood, mostly toward the end of his life, the tenor of his language changes, and the man who once was the New Testament's most fiery preacher finds an internal space of contentedness and peace. From a prison cell in Rome, he writes what many biblical scholars consider his last epistle, declaring,

> I have learned to be content whatever the circumstances. I know what it is to be in need, and I know what it is to have plenty. I have *learned the secret* of being content in any and every situation, whether well fed or hungry, whether living in plenty or in want. I can do all this through him who gives me strength.[1]

Though he has every reason to worry about his circumstance, complain about his lack of comfort or companionship, and doubt the very God whom he has so faithfully served, Paul instead speaks of the wellness of his soul. The warrior and king we have witnessed throughout the scripture have somehow come to rest in that Roman cell. I believe the secret Paul speaks of here is a result of his transition into his second-half Sage.

THE SECRET

There is a holy settledness in the heart of the Sage that comes not only from a lifetime of experience but also from an absorption of God's grace and goodness along the way. Paul tells us, "I have learned the secret," and then he points to the strength of spirit found in the Lord himself. He guides us to a sacred acceptance that life here on earth will never fulfill all our needs, dreams, or desires, and yet a deeper hope exists beyond this world. He is grounded, aware, and willing to receive whatever God may bring, his wisdom leading us to the true and deeper well. Rather than turn the volume up on his apostolic calling, we see Paul descend to a place of peace and well-being. It is as if he knows something beyond knowing.

Jesus also playfully invites his disciples to a deeper knowing. In Luke 12, he instructs:

> Therefore I tell you, do not worry about your life, what you will eat; or about your body, what you will wear. For life is more than food, and the body more than clothes. Consider the ravens: They do not sow or reap, they have no storeroom or barn; yet God feeds them. And how much more valuable you are than birds! Who of you by worrying can add a single hour to your life? Since you cannot do this very little thing, why do you worry about the rest?
>
> Consider how the wildflowers grow. They do not labor or spin. Yet I tell you, not even Solomon in all his splendor was dressed like one of these. If that is how God clothes the grass of the field, which is here today, and tomorrow is thrown into the fire, how much more will he clothe you—you of little faith! And do not set your heart on what you will eat or drink; do not worry about it. For the pagan world runs after all such things, and your Father knows that you need them. But seek his kingdom, and these things will be given to you as well.[2]

"Do not worry," Jesus says. God knows what you need. Calm down and be well, friends. Be well.

And yet here we are, spending most of our lives as men worrying about the things we have or don't have, and how much. Our possessions consume us; we worry about our reputations; and we fear our unknown futures. Most men are completely unfamiliar with contentment. It is true, God invites us to co-labor with him in stewarding our resources and tending to the needs of our families and communities. But in this passage, Jesus reorients our hearts away from materialism, hedonism, and narcissism toward the kingdom, and he opens our eyes to the great benevolence of the loving Father.

As we become Sages, it is vital for us to join Paul's descent into this reality and settle into the contentment of the Lord. Rohr tells us, "Your concern is not so much *to have what you love* anymore, but *to love what you have*–right now. This is a monumental change from the first half of life, so much so that it is almost the litmus test of whether you are in the second half of life at all."[3]

The Sage of the second half has moved away from the constant drive for bigger and better and finds joy in the gift of the present. It truly is the secret.

A few summers ago, on a Restoration Project father-daughter backpacking trip,[4] our team hiked up the steep edge of the Continental Divide and began the descent down the other side. I had the great fortune of taking my own daughter, Sophie, on that trek, along with my friends Bart and Shae and their two daughters. Once past the loose scree and the steep, knee-buckling switchbacks, we descended into a high alpine meadow where the stunning beauty took our breath away. There, close to 11,000 feet, on a rarely traveled trail, the glory of Jesus's words from Luke came alive. The green grasses of the meadow danced in the cool breeze while a million wildflowers raised their glorious faces in praise towards the sky: yellow, white, purple, pink, red, and blue. Bees hopped from bud to bud, and the tops of the trees swayed as if waving their hands in unison with the song below. A few of us stopped, hypnotized by the rapturous view, while the Spirit of God whispered softly in our ears, "*Consider how the wild flowers grow...*"

I will never forget Bart's wise words once we caught our collective breath: "Oh, the extravagant waste of God. Here we are in this remote place, and God's greatness and goodness crafted and created each one of these flowers for his own delight and pleasure. It's his grace to allow our little group to stumble upon them today. And maybe he made them just for us to see. But how many meadows, how many flowers exist *right now* that no human eye will ever see? The abundance of God is so great, he has enough to waste extravagantly in meadows like this and on people like us."

Bart, my fellow second-half journeyman, is beginning to know Paul's secret too.

It is this same knowing I caught wind of as a teenager, standing at the split-rail fence with Ben. As he looked out over the mountains, I knew he felt the tempest swirling inside of me. But it did not scare him. It did not fluster him. He remained unmoved–not unfeeling, but *unmoved*. He offered no advice on how to navigate it, no expert words of what I should do or not do. He just stood there–present, kind, and *with* me in such a way I could anchor myself to him. He knew something I desperately wanted to know. As a tall, broad mountain man, he possessed a fair amount of muscle, but it was not this physical strength that calmed me. It was the strength of his being, the gravity of his presence, and the grounded contentedness of his soul. He knew Paul's secret and invited me to borrow from him while I slowly learned it for myself over the next several decades. Since then, I have returned to that fence a thousand times in my mind, just to live for another moment inside the settled contentedness of a Sage I once knew.

For so long, I lived from a posture of scarcity. Though I had my physical needs met as a child, so many of my emotional and relational needs remained unseen and missed. I learned quickly and early how to survive in this emotional desert, picking my way through the debris in an attempt to find enough scraps to feed my soul. As I grew into adulthood, this scrappiness came with me, and the fear of not having enough fueled the drive to avoid hunger at all costs. I learned how to keep my distance from relationships, having lost hope that any soul food might be available to me. I learned to prefer distance over potential disappointment, and I found ways to scrounge together my own relational meals rather than wonder if God might provide for me there. Contentedness felt ever elusive, and, like most men, I barely dipped my toes in its soothing waters. To move closer to the Sage, however, I had to settle my younger scrappy self and lean into the secret of God's great provision.

One of the first hallmarks of a second-half Sage is his settled contentment, which presents as a holy satisfaction. He has come to accept himself, his world, his role, and his circumstances for the gifts they are, not what he hoped they would be. His striving has ceased, and he welcomes the moment for what it brings. In the first half of our lives, we "put our inner lives on hold, devaluing contact with the sacred in favor of mastering the skills needed in the everyday utilitarian world. [But the second half] gives us the opportunity to reconnect with the sacred dimension of life."[5] As a Sage, we learn the definition of *enoughness* and live from a posture of gratitude and awe rather than the never-ending pursuit for more. Our eyes are open to the ever-present sacred, and we have enough inner stillness to seek the kingdom found in everything and everyone.

Descending the Continental Divide, I noticed only a few of us paused to take in the majesty of the meadow. Most of the group continued marching forward, eyes watching the rocky trail, bodies ready to make camp after such a strenuous climb. The promise of lakes and food and the thought of setting down their 40-pound packs drove them right past the Edenic splendor. And while they did make it to camp first, they also missed a fantastic display of the extravagant wastefulness of God.

ENOUGH

One of the many challenges my intellectually disabled sister faces is *hyperphagia*, a disorder caused by Prader-Willi syndrome, in which her body's cues to determine her stomach's fullness remain permanently offline. Simply put, she has no measure of her appetite and will continue to eat until someone stops her or she gets physically sick. Throughout her life, this has caused a variety of gastrointestinal problems, as well as a consistent struggle with maintaining a healthy weight and blood chemistry. Though she is half my physical stature, she could out-eat me any day.

As a result, my parents often talked about *being full*. "Are you full?" they asked us as children. Or my mother would declare, "You kids have had *enough*." My father, on the other hand, used the word differently, regularly coming to the end of his patience and gruffly barking, "That's *enough!*" As a boy, I rarely knew what enough looked like or felt like on my own, always wondering when the imaginary and seemingly arbitrary line would be crossed. Enough seemed to carry a negative tone, and I learned to keep my distance at an early age.

However, as an exchange student in high school learning a new language, I discovered a new and deeper sense of what "full" and "enough" might mean. I love how learning new languages helps us understand our own native tongues more deeply. One evening at dinner early in my year abroad, my German host mother generously offered me a second pork chop. Honored by her kind offer but not enthusiastic about her cooking, I quickly translated in my head, *Nein danke, ich bin voll.* "No, thank you. I am full."

She smiled at the slightly awkward use of the word *voll*. "Chris," she said patiently in slow and enunciated German, "glasses are full of water, trains are full of people, suitcases are full of clothes, but people are not full."

Embarrassed by my mistake, I responded, "What are people then?"

Leute sind zufrieden. People are satisfied.

In that moment, not only did she teach me a new German word and its proper use, she taught me an entirely new concept: satisfaction. To be satisfied is not an absence of desire, hunger, or appetite. It is not, as many men have been instructed, the *killing of desire*[6], but rather it is the fulfillment of it. In order for a desire to be satisfied, it must first exist, be listened and attended to, and then met with careful particularity. As Christian men, we have been taught to say no to desire, learning to fear it, avoid it, and suppress it, when in fact we must collectively reimagine what it means to say a holy and God-filled " yes!" God gave us desires he means to satisfy.

> To be satisfied is not an absence of desire, hunger, or appetite. It is not, as many men have been instructed, the killing of desire, but rather it is the fulfillment of it.

Often, we attempt to satisfy our desire with things we do not actually want. We have not attuned to it, listened to it, or wondered about it long enough to seek out the particular means by which to satisfy it. The hole in our hearts calls for *something,* and we run to quench the thirst before we wonder what it is thirsty for. With the slightest pangs of such desire, we stand in front of the proverbial refrigerator with the door open, looking for a snack to feed our soul. As a father, I cannot count the number of times my young children said, "Dad, I'm hungry," quickly grabbing a bag of potato chips or Cheez-Its from the pantry. It drove me insane, knowing much of the time they were not hungry at all but turned to chips when they were bored, lonely, or needed a break. As with most issues in fathering, parenting them forced me to look inward, and my annoyance broke when I recognized how often I stood staring into the metaphorical pantry myself. When we feed our hearts unsubstantial food, we will never truly be satisfied. Bluntly stated, novelist Bruce Marshall states, "The young man who rings the bell at the brothel is unconsciously looking for God."[7] We are not truly hungry for the things we end up feeding our hearts.

The quest for more is woven into the fabric of the American dream. More money, more days off, more sales, more authority, more profit, more impact. The insatiable pursuit exists in all spheres, including, and maybe especially, in the Church. More pews, more donations, more converts, more baptisms, more downloads, more members...the list goes on. As Christopher West writes, many men try "to suck infinity out of finite things. But finite things...can never satisfy our yearning for the infinite. Once I've attained what I thought I wanted but I'm still left wanting, what do I think I need? *More.* Then when I attain more and it still doesn't satisfy me, what do I think I need? *More* and *more* and *more...*"[8] The true antithesis of *enough* is *more*. As a people, we have satisfaction amnesia. We have forgotten what it means to be *zufrieden*. Interestingly, *zu-frieden* literally translates to *at peace*.

The Sage discovers the expansive inner space of contentedness when he learns to listen to his desires, recognizes God's ultimate provision for them, and makes peace with them. He notices them, feeds them, loves them, and tends to them with the care of a master gardener, not under- or over-watering them with too little or too much, for both lead to death. He meets his desire with enough, and there unearths his peace. He has learned to sit in the painful tension between his infinite desire and his temporary existence in a finite world. He

> ...allows himself to feel the deepest depths of human desire and chooses to 'stay in the pain' of wanting more than this life has to offer...He is able to both do without the many pleasures of this world *and* to rejoice in all the true pleasures of this world without idolizing them—that is, without trying to suck infinity out of them.[9]

This is what the Apostle Paul calls us to as he sits with *enough* in his Roman prison cell. He may not have all he needs, but he has found the territory of enough.

The Psalmist invites us to a similar place:

Lord, you alone are my portion and my cup; you make my lot secure.
   The boundary lines have fallen for me in pleasant places; surely I have a delightful inheritance.
   I will praise the Lord, who counsels me; even at night my heart instructs me.
   I keep my eyes always on the Lord.
   With him at my right hand, I will not be shaken.

> *Therefore my heart is glad and my tongue rejoices; my body also will rest secure, because you will not abandon me to the realm of the dead, nor will you let your faithful one see decay.*
>
> *You make known to me the path of life; you will fill me with joy in your presence, with eternal pleasures at your right hand.*[10]

The pursuit of enough does not depend on our own scrappiness to provide but on our recognition of the provision of God, who himself is our "portion." He is not too little, nor is he too much. He is our enough. He has set our boundary lines, not us, and though we may seek to expand our lands and increase our domain, he is the one who has established what is ours and what is not. The Sage accepts his existence, including his passions, desires, and dreams, as a foreshadowing of the glory and kingdom to come. He recognizes with the Psalmist, "I remain confident of this: I will see the goodness of the Lord in the land of the living."[11] In this confidence, the Sage finds peace.

Many men I know live as practical atheists in this regard, spending their lives in the insatiable pursuit of more. They live as if *they* are the ones to secure their lives and *they* are the determiners of their "portion." Of the limited resources in the world, *they* must secure their share. Rather than constantly keeping their eyes on the unshakable God, they find themselves discontent and rattled when Wall Street quivers, a competitor launches a brilliant new product, a new church plant opens down the street, or the arbitrarily set revenue goal is not met. Only the infinite can satisfy infinite desire. Clearly, *zufrieden* remains a foreign concept, and satisfaction is an ever-alluring fantasy.

I am not an unambitious man nor exempt from this struggle. No one can accuse me of laziness, and more often than not, my friends, coworkers, and counselors tell me to slow down. When Ben, the Sage from the split-rail fence, performed our wedding, he said of me, "Chris has two gears: full speed ahead and full stop." He is right. I love the thrill of accomplishment just as much as the next guy. I engage most tasks as if they were designed to challenge my grit and capacity, and I am determined to prove them wrong. And then, when it is time to rest, I cherish long quiet days of nothingness, and my wife claims I fall asleep in seconds.

As such, I have regularly wrestled the dichotomy between resignation and consumption, two opposing poles on the spectrum of enoughness.[12] On one end burns the fire of demand, a battle-frenzy pursuit of the ever-elusive "next thing." It is sought out, achieved, consumed, and then quickly forgotten as the corner is turned and new prospects appear. On the other end lies the cold winterland of abdication, where effort and attempt are meaningless and the snooze button, doom-scrolling, and "whatever" develop into close companions. Somewhere between these two extremes we find both true desire and true enough. We find peace. Ambition, desire, and contentedness are not at odds. In fact, they are terrific companions when reimagined in light of the enoughness of God.

The Sage has come to reside in the realm of enough. Whether big or small, plenty or simple, the internal posture of his heart says, "It is enough for today." Akin to Jesus in John 4 after he speaks with the woman at the well and the disciples return from the village with lunch, the Sage eats from an entirely different table. As does Jesus. He refuses earthly food and says, "I have food to eat that you know nothing about….My food is to do the will of him who sent me and to finish his work."[13] It is here the man finds what his scrappy boy needs.

A Sage is first known by his settled contentment, which opens an increasingly vast space inside the territory of his soul. From contentment, he now grows a spacious inner hospitality to welcome others into his uncrowded heart.

———

QUESTIONS TO CONSIDER AND DISCUSS:

- *What is your experience of zufrieden? What does it mean to you to be satisfied?*
- *What do you know of your own "scrappy boy?" How have you had to provide for your own needs, whether physically, emotionally, psychologically, or spiritually?*
- *How would you describe your "enough?" How do you know when you have enough?*
- *What anxiety do you have with regard to God's extravagant waste?*
- *Review your contentedness. Where are you settled? Where are you not?*

11

THE SAGE'S WELCOME: A SPACIOUS INNER HOSPITALITY

As a business owner and ministry leader, I am regularly invited to participate in and/or speak at various networking and luncheon events. Due to the nature of my work with men, most of these invitations come from men's groups with older men who have found community in these spaces. These guys have participated in their communities for decades, often serving on nonprofit boards, city councils, or school boards and volunteering their expertise in times of crisis or need. They are generally good-hearted men.

Several years ago, I received an invitation to eat breakfast with some like-minded men and share about Restoration Project. I was told I would have 20 minutes to introduce our work before the meal and then an opportunity to answer questions as they arose. The whole event would be no more than an hour, as the meeting took place at the start of the work day and many needed to hurry off by 8 a.m.

Though billed as a "businessman's" gathering, the group met in a large, sterile, cinder-block room at an old downtown church. A few round tables surrounded by folding chairs sat like islands in the vast room, and a 60-year-old lectern with a telescoping microphone stood resolutely at the front, ready for the day's presentations. I arrived a few minutes early to meet the host, orient myself to the space, and settle in.

Three hours later, I drove away, stifled, dismissed, and enraged.

After a 30-minute introduction and welcome to all attendees by the emcee (there were 20 men, and I was the only newcomer), the chapter chairman took another 30 minutes to share about the birth of his newest grandson, the good work the city golf course was doing to keep the greens clear of goose droppings, and the upcoming charity event he hoped everyone would attend. The first hour came and went.

The breakfast buffet opened, so we broke the program to eat pancakes and bacon, accompanied by chit-chat around the tables. Once the emcee finished his coffee, he returned to the podium and announced our program for the day, which included an ecological report about a new solar program, a retirement celebration for a long-standing member, and a speech from the CEO of Restoration Project (i.e. me). Second hour, gone. By the time I spoke, half the attendees had left to get to work, and the remaining men sat disinterested. Needless to say, my comments were brief, giving only a cursory fly-over of our work, knowing that by that point, everyone was ready to leave. Though the room was full of older men, it felt void of Sages.

The second great hallmark of the second-half Sage is his generous and spacious hospitality. This of course includes his *actual* hospitality, where he welcomes you into his home, office, or environment, taking care to attend to your comfort and care. In fact, the Sage's actual physical space itself is designed with the guest in mind, anticipating his arrival and preparing for his presence.

The other form of hospitality is the *internal* space the second-half man has to welcome you. He knows what space he occupies in the world and holds that space solidly and stalwartly. Like a lighthouse on the shore, he stands firm and strong whether in sun or storm. He has done the deep work of creating an inner home for himself. He is no longer worried about where he belongs because he now belongs to himself. Together with his settled contentedness, he possesses an inner sanctuary in which he finds rest. As he enters this peace, others can as well. The key here is that he occupies his space, and no more. He no longer needs to prove himself to anyone, and he does not need to be the most important person in the room. As one Sage puts it, "There can only be room within my office for another if I make room, if I cease to occupy enough space so that the other can come in, not dissolved before my power and authority but encased in his own atmosphere."[1] Hospitality requires us to make emotional, psychological, mental, and spiritual space for others to enter and find a place to sit.

Neither external nor internal space was offered to me at that men's gathering. Rather than create space, the men consumed it, thereby creating an atmosphere where no one but they could exist. I know this group does good things for our community, but it is not a spaciously hospitable group. It's a first-half space full of elderly men.

Throughout the first half, we are conditioned to take up space, make more of ourselves, develop and grow and fill. We ascend the ladders of influence, authority, and leadership, making our way to our version of the throne room where our importance is venerated and our words are heeded. Or, like squatters in our unoccupied inner territory, we allow others unhindered access to our lives, mortgaging our space in the hopes of favor, security, and earned privilege. First-half men focus on the increase of their power, not their decrease. Even our language describes this. We are *promoted, climb the ladder,* and *rise to the top*. As we increase, so does our "seniority," and we have bigger budgets, bigger offices, bigger staffs, and bigger egos. Our narcissism is fanned into flame, and we are trained to always want more.

THE REWARD FOR NARCISSISM

My boss and I arrived at the campus of a large, well-known ministry headquarters a few minutes early in order to find the right building, check in, get our "visitor" badges, and await further instructions. We drove past the bookstore featuring thousands of resources this ministry has produced over the years and noticed the parking lot was already full of patrons waiting for the doors to open at 10 a.m. Though I wondered how we would find the correct building amongst the dozens on their campus, my co-pilot, himself the president of a well-known ministry, simply said, "Look for the biggest and most opulent edifice. That'll be the one." He was right.

Our meeting with the president and CEO of this ministry had been on the calendar for several months now. The producers of their popular radio station heard about one of my colleague's books and wanted to feature him on the show. But first, in order to adequately "vet" him, the president needed to speak with him.

We waited in the second floor lobby, akin to the antechamber of the Oval Office, with blue carpet, limited-access badges, American flags flanking the reception desk, and the ministry's insignia and vision statement boldly emblazoned on the wall. Ten minutes after our scheduled appointment, an intern with a tablet fetched us, escorting us through the locked double doors into a large boardroom, complete with a 20-foot table and seven chairs on each side. He told us to "sit here" as he pointed to the middle seats on one side of the table. Obediently, we took our places and waited another several minutes, soft worship music playing in the background.

Without warning, a side door opened, and six identically dressed and smiling middle-aged white men with leather-bound notepads entered the room. As if on cue, each man unbuttoned his blue blazer, flattened his tie, and sat in one of the seven chairs opposite us. They saved the middle seat for the last of their parade, the esteemed president and CEO, who likewise entered the room with a smile and a greeting as he took his seat. After each man introduced himself in order of importance, making sure to include their position titles and years of service, the president turned his attention to us and said, "Great to meet you, and thanks for coming. But I'm sorry, *who* are you?"

Adept and wise Sage that he is, my colleague navigated the pomp and pretense of the next 37 minutes with ninja-like skill. Designed to intimidate, the seven-on-two setup meant to communicate the significance of the ministry's success and especially the prowess and power of the president who led them to achieve it. Unknowingly, we stepped into the fantasy world of a culture committed to uphold the narcissism of its leader. Personal identities had been put aside, and the exaltation of the one had become the focus. Though each of the six supporting actors asked questions and jotted down notes, it was clear no one's thoughts or opinions would be consulted in making the final decision.

Ultimately, the radio interview was granted, and the entourage departed with the same ceremony with which they entered. We were left to find our way out. As we made our way back to our car, my colleague and I could barely contain our laughter and expletives. We had just witnessed a great display of narcissistic theater, and we were dying. In fact, by the time we reached our vehicle, we erupted at the hilarity of it all to such a degree other visitors likely wondered about our sanity.

What I experienced that day sits at the top of my engagements with narcissism, and yet there are a thousand lesser degrees with which we all regularly contend. In the eyes of the world and even in the eyes of the American church, as evidenced by this ministry leader, we laud those who ascend to great levels of leadership and succeed widely in the advancement of their ministry's mission and impact. As businessmen, ministers, and men in general, we are validated for our increase and instructed to always strive to be the most important person around.

Our narcissism is rewarded, and in a self-perpetuating cycle, our ego grows and fills more of the room around us. We explain it away and spiritualize it with internal dialogue that says, "For such a time as this" or "God has given me 10 talents to steward" or "God continues to bless our work." While it is true we are called to co-labor with God in the subduing of the earth and the advancement of his name and kingdom, far too often we lose him in the process. We become addicted to the accolades, benefits, and how good it feels to be needed and wanted, allowing our narcissism to grow unchecked. In my own journey, I have known this path all too well.

All of us are narcissists to some degree. Each and every one. We all fall in love with the sight of our own face and the sound of our own voice. We pursue our self-interest and find ways to advance our own name and agenda. Narcissism is part of the human experience and has been since the beginning. Inside each of us is a scared little boy who fears *who he is* simply cannot be sufficient, loved, or accepted; therefore, he finds ways to puff out his chest and take up more space. His fear drives him to believe he must become bigger and more in order to be welcome. As we move further into the second half, however, we must be keenly aware of our self-importance and especially awake to how others feel in our presence.

While you may not have experienced a narcissistic boardroom such as the one I described,[2] you likely have plenty of examples of more subtle or covert narcissism. You may know what it feels like to have a conversation with someone, only arriving at the end of your time desperate to end his monologue. You may know how it feels to be missed, not heard, not pursued, and then blamed for being too quiet or protected. You may have the experience of losing yourself in the well-woven tales and visions of an inspirational leader, and even offer yourself in service of his plan, only to walk away realizing how much of your soul you just mortgaged. You might know those men about whom everyone else says, "He's great! Such a great guy!" and yet when you spend time with him, he tells you all about himself and waits until the last five minutes of the time to ask, "So, how are *you*?" These are just a few examples of the daily narcissism we encounter.

To be clear, narcissism is not born of arrogance but from fear. It emerges in the soul in those young moments of wounding when we experience abandonment, loss, and neglect. Terrified of being overlooked, left, or dismissed, our egos compensate by elevating ourselves and diminishing others. We inflate our self-importance to avoid our shame.

And yet, the paradoxical way of Jesus points us to the inverse. To have life is to lose it. To be first we must be last. To reign is to serve. To be the king of the universe is to arrive on earth in an out-of-the-way backwater stable, not in the opulence of a golden tower. Though our narcissism is rewarded throughout our first half of life, a significant indicator of a man's intentional movement over the threshold into his second half is the degree to which he divests of his ego's need for elevation and instead finds his way back to the dirt. Like John the Baptist, he says, "He must become greater; I must become less."[3] Or as Proverbs 26:12 warns, "Do you see a man wise in his own eyes? There is more hope for a fool than for him."[4] We must confront our inner narcissist, repent of our addiction to our own self-importance and self-advancement, and bring our ego back in check. Only then can we create within ourselves a generous hospitality that welcomes the other with enough space for him to exist without contending with our overwhelming presence. This requires years of internal work to re-integrate our true selves with the selves we thought we needed to be. And as with all things in the kingdom, there is always more awareness, more repentance, more grace, and more healing to be had in reseating the True King on the throne of our hearts.

> We must confront our inner narcissist, repent of our addiction to our own self-importance and self-advancement, and bring our ego back in check.

LOSING YOURSELF TO CREATE SPACE FOR OTHERS

As we divest ourselves of our masks, re-collect our projections, and integrate the wisdom from each stage of our masculine journey, we are free to see beyond ourselves, diminish our greatness, and welcome the stranger into our midst. Again, we follow Paul's descending journey as he refuses to boast in his accomplishments and instead counts them as worthless trash compared to his settledness in Christ. Consider Paul's words to the church in Philippi:

> *If someone else thinks they have reasons to put confidence in the flesh, I have more: circumcised on the eighth day, of the people of Israel, of the tribe of Benjamin, a Hebrew of Hebrews; in regard to the law, a Pharisee; as for zeal, persecuting the church; as for righteousness based on the law, faultless. But whatever were gains to me I now consider loss for the sake of Christ.*
>
> *What is more, I consider everything a loss because of the surpassing worth of knowing Christ Jesus my Lord, for whose sake I have lost all things. I consider them garbage, that I may gain Christ and be found in him, not having a righteousness of my own that comes from the law, but that which is through faith in Christ—the righteousness that comes from God on the basis of faith.*[5]

In the world of the Hebrews, Paul has every reason to boast. Both his lineage and his education provide him position and privilege, yet he casts them aside in a passionate pursuit of Christ.

Unfortunately, many men do not make this downward journey but instead consider their achievements, titles, and acquisitions to be the very reason they *should* have a pedestal on which to stand. Their worth and meaning continue to be rooted in their wealth, whether financial gains, expansive influence, or expert knowledge. Throughout my life, when I have consulted older men for wisdom, rarely have I sought their expertise or advice. The world is full of experts. As John Eldredge points out,

The sage, on the other hand, communes with God—an existence entirely different from and utterly superior to the life of the expert. Whatever counsel he offers, he draws you to God, not to self-reliance....[The Sage] offers a gift of presence, the richness of a soul that has lived long *with* God.[6]

Rather than advice or expertise, what I have needed from Sages is their hospitality to a younger man who longs to be seen and offered a steadfast hand amid life's storms.

In some streams of Jewish philosophy, we find the concept of *tzimtzum*. In literal terms, this means *contraction* or *drawing back*. When considering the creation of the world by an omnipresent and all-powerful God, Jewish thought reasons that in order to create something other, something not-God, he "drew back the infinite to create a space in which finitude could be realized."[7] As an illustrative example, imagine Mozart teaching an elementary school music class. For students to comprehend the basics of scores and notes, he would have to *draw back* and put aside all his musical abilities in complex symphonic composition. He would not lose them, forget them, or become less Mozart, but by drawing himself back, he creates space for the younger learners to be where they are in their educational and musical journey, not his.

In a similar way, the second-half man may have an abundance of thought, experience, perspective, and expertise he could offer another man 20 or 30 years his junior. But in order to create space, in order to be truly hospitable to the other, he *draws back*. He has come to realize his life is not about him. He has nothing more to prove and nothing more to gain. He needs nothing of the other man, but instead, he can offer a spacious presence that creates rather than demands. One Sage says, "On the human level, withdrawal of myself aids the other to come into being."[8] When a man is able to withdraw and yet remain near, others find solid ground on which they can plant their feet.

This does not require the Sage to become any less important or powerful. Remember, the most powerful character in every hero's journey is not the hero himself, but the guide, the Sage. We all know the most revered and feared character in *The Lord of the Rings* is Gandalf. The most venerated Jedi Master in *Star Wars* is Yoda, and the most powerful wizard in the magical world of *Harry Potter* is Professor Dumbledore. What is most remarkable, however, is how much space each of these Sages creates for those around him and how that space is the foundation on which the emerging heroes actually become the heroes they are. When the Sage can tend to his own internal, scared little boy, he has space to care for others as well.

As I write while retreating on the far western coast of the Dingle Peninsula of Ireland, just down the street is Kruger's Bar, venerated as "the most westerly pub in Europe." There are very few people in these far reaches of the galaxy and very few historical moments by which this sleepy little Irish village can claim fame. However, surprising to the visitor merely seeking a pint, on Kruger's wall hangs a plaque and several photographs of Chewbacca.

Upon closer inspection, I learn significant portions of the 2017 blockbuster *Star Wars: The Last Jedi* were filmed along this very coast. The rugged terrain and steep cliffs, along with the constantly wet weather, seemed the perfect place to locate Master Luke's secret Jedi hideaway island. The crew built the set for the Jedi's refuge and temple, and then they disassembled it upon completion of the project. Visitors today only see roadside placards pointing to the locations of the shoot. They are the only road signs for miles.

Naturally, in solidarity with my local hosts, I re-watch the film, though this time, I pay special attention to Master Yoda. Throughout the story, though his part is relatively minor, I am again struck by his unflappable nature and his spacious generosity. In this and previous movies, he waits, observes, and allows the drama to unfold. He is kind yet firm, and he asks questions rather than offers advice. His patience with Luke's petulance is astounding, and he merely grunts under his breath and slowly closes his eyes with an awareness that says, "I knew that petulance inside me once too." In one scene, the ancient, sacred Jedi texts are in danger of being consumed by fire. While Luke desperately attempts to save them, Yoda merely jokes, "Page turners, they were not." This Master Jedi is settled, knowing what he knows and allowing Luke to borrow from his space. Only then does Luke become Yoda's counterpart.

To be such a Sage requires one to be at home with himself, to know his purpose, meaning, and place in this world. Nouwen says, "It requires first of all that the host feel at home in his own house, and secondly that he creates a free and fearless place for the unexpected visitor."[9] If a man remains unsettled and at war with himself, his own ego, and his own scared younger self, then he cannot be a second-half man. He must integrate and absorb the wisdom of the first half before he can offer this spacious hospitality to another. Otherwise, though he may be full of experience and knowledge, all he can offer is advice and expertise as a means to justify his life's accomplishments and ego's importance. Again, Eldredge says it well:

> It is a matter of presence. A sage does not have to be heard, as a warrior might, does not have to rule, as a king might. There is room in his presence for who you are and where you are. There is understanding. He has no agenda, and nothing now to lose. What he offers, he offers with kindness, and discretion.[10]

There is space inside the Sage for others to find rest.

The first hallmark of the Sage is his settled contentedness, which then creates within him an inner spacious hospitality for others. As he welcomes the stranger, his generous spirituality is such that he can offer his guests the freedom to break from the tight binds of black and white, either/or perspectives, considering with them the possibility that the Great Story may be larger and our Great God may be kinder than we ever imagined.

QUESTIONS TO CONSIDER AND DISCUSS:

- *What experiences have you had of men who considered themselves more important than others? How was that for you?*
- *In what ways has narcissism been rewarded in your life?*
- *What fear drives a person to puff up and self-aggrandize? How can you have empathy for that younger part in others and in yourself?*
- *What does it feel like to be in the presence of a Sage who has spacious hospitality to offer you?*

12

THE SAGE'S GREAT GOD: GENEROUS SPIRITUALITY

As a young and newly married man, I found great delight and comfort in knowing all I could about God, doctrine, and the Scripture. Both my wife and I read voraciously, and nerdy as it sounds, we often found ourselves reading for hours in the evenings of our first year together. We lived in Chicago and made very little money in our first jobs after college, so we quickly solidified our identities as bibliophiles by acquainting ourselves with the thousands of free books at the public library. For our first anniversary we decided a celebration was in order, planning and penny-pinching our way west. To *Iowa*. While not the typical first anniversary destination for a young couple, our travel- and adventure-hungry selves found a German-style hotel, complete with the timber and beam *fachwerk* I had come to love as an exchange student in high school. After seeing pictures of the building's "library," we grew excited and set out on our Midwest adventure. Now, 27 years later, we look back at our younger selves with a smile, a chuckle, and a "bless you, young people!" under our breath.

On this particular road trip, Beth and I did something no other young couple has ever done for fun–we read *out loud* to each other

Wayne Grudem's newly released *Systematic Theology*.[1] We reveled in the careful articulation of complicated biblical concepts and solidified our theological foundations with logic and truth. Now that our university studies were complete, we turned our full academic attention to the pursuit of knowing God. Having both become Christians in high school, and with faith stories more akin to spiritual meandering than any sort of rootedness in a church denomination or tradition, our theological interests were broad but not deep. Sinking our intellectual teeth into the structure of Grudem's well-articulated doctrinal positions, we felt our young faith settling into a spiritual home. Later, when we launched into international missions, we intentionally chose one of the world's hardest mission fields, convinced not to waste our lives with what might be easier, more comfortable, or borderline hedonistic.[2] At our core, we are a principled couple, and early on, we dedicated our lives to the kingdom with everything we had. Bless us. Today, if you ask me about it, you may get a major eye roll.

THE SAFETY OF FIRST HALF KNOWING

As a young man, I needed to know without a doubt the crystal-clear right and wrong, yes and no, truth and lie. I needed a biblical structure that had sound and convincing logic and could easily answer my toughest theological questions. I also needed a God I could understand, a God who fit into boxes with axioms I could not only grasp but also argue and articulate to those around me. I found incredible relief in Grudem's well-organized gospel and wholeheartedly surrendered myself to a systematized faith.

Right around this time, Luis Bush, the CEO of Partners International, an organization sending missionaries around the globe, coined the term *10/40 Window*, referring to the portion of the world framed by 10- and 40-degrees north latitude. His research showed that within this box, reaching from North Africa through the Middle East and into the Far East, lived the world's largest populations suffering from severe poverty *and* the least access to Christian resources.³ Rallied by the call to "reach the world for Christ," thousands of young missionaries joined the movement and headed overseas.

The 10/40 Window gave me the missiological clarity I needed by identifying the "lost." It provided for us a yes and no, an us and them, a group of people who needed access to Jesus. It solidified a well-defined goal for my passionate heart, and the Zealous Warrior within me saw past my job in finance at Campbell's Soup and found the mountain I believed I was designed, impassioned, and purposed to conquer: to bring Christ to the 10/40 Window.

Armed with this clear vision and this systematized approach to God, Beth and I set out to evangelize the world for Christ. I was the ripe old age of 24. Again, I bless that younger man for his clarity, purpose, and zeal.

THE GREAT UNKNOWING

In the journey of my late 20s and early 30s, however, when the ground of the mission field proved too hard to penetrate and the "missionary graveyard" claimed more and more of my teammates with depression, anxiety, or burnout, my rigid belief system felt increasingly anemic. The goodness of God seemed to slowly dissipate, the bright hope of the kingdom seemed to wane, and something inside me shifted. The solidity of my theological formulas started to wobble, and the questions my experience forced me to ask suddenly had insufficient answers. The Bible and its systematic rules no longer made sense, and I found myself stumbling and faltering over the theology in which I had once found such comfort and clarity. What I lived out on the international mission field felt far more gray than the black and white of my Chicago suburbs, and I had no categories for what I now faced.

My time in the 10/40 Window tested my beliefs in ways only pain, suffering, and grief can. I watched several colleagues spin out and leave the field, some closer to atheism than to Jesus upon their departure. I witnessed many converts or near-converts struggle with the cost of "becoming a Christian" far more than what it meant to follow Jesus, for to convert their religion meant to disown not only their families but their heritage and homeland as well. As Lewis says,

> You never know how much you really believe anything until its truth or falsehood becomes a matter of life and death to you. It is easy to say you believe a rope to be strong and sound as long as you are merely using it to cord a box. But suppose you had to hang by that rope over a precipice. Wouldn't you then first discover how much you really trusted it?[4]

While my faith in Jesus deepened during this time, my trust in the theological rope diminished as I watched far too many of my dear friends fall off the cliff.

I had come to the end of the spiritual box I had so painstakingly crafted in my early 20s. Rather than the concrete yes or no I had come to hold so dear, I learned about God's in-between, his willingness to step outside human systems to recover my heart. And your heart. And their hearts. Apparently, God refuses to be boxed.

Over the next several years, I wrestled with the constructs with which I had indoctrinated myself. I wondered at the darkness of my own heart and marveled at the transformation blessing invited over judgment. I saw the edges of my own soul turn towards depression as futility and exhaustion ebbed ever nearer. I sought psychological help and began taking medication. Though still principled and committed to the advancement of the kingdom, my theology wore down to a nub, and my faith shattered into a million pieces. Thankfully and by God's grace, "my idea of God is not a divine idea. It has to be shattered time after time. He shatters it Himself."[5] I grew closer to Jesus and away from systems. Through this dark season, Jesus invited me to a new space, one I had vehemently rejected as a younger man. It was the unboxed space of the in-between.

The possibility emerged for me to be both a faithful believer and follower of Jesus while still doubting significantly. Somehow I learned to hold the truth of God's goodness and restoration in one hand while recognizing significant pain, loss, and senseless suffering in the other. Both had to coexist. My ideas and experience of God grew beyond the confines of the box, and his immensity in my eyes grew all the more.

For many men like me, this is an extremely challenging transition. It shakes the very foundations on which we base our lives, loves, ministries, and decisions. For some, it calls into question the very definition of what it means to be a Christian and confronts our notion of church and God. In order to pass the threshold of the second half, however, we must turn from our firm commitment to boxes and defined lines and welcome a God who is unwilling to be confined by our limited understanding. As God says through the prophet Isaiah, "For my thoughts are not your thoughts, neither are your ways my ways…As the heavens are higher than the earth, so are my ways higher than your ways, and my thoughts than your thoughts."[6] Second-half Sages move toward the mystery of God, not away, and welcome God's victory over their first-half theological egos.

> Second-half Sages move toward the mystery of God, not away, and welcome God's victory over their first-half theological egos.

THE DOWNWARD JOURNEY OF SECOND-HALF SPIRITUALITY

Now, some 20 years later and at this midlife juncture of my life, I recognize I have merely started to read the preface of God's Great Story, barely beginning to know the depths of who God is and who I am in Him. This can only begin to be explored in my lifetime. I might be tempted to look back on the younger man I once was, the man who thought he "understood" God, with a shameful scoff and an eye roll. We are all idolaters after all, constructing the images of God we believe to be the most true, right, and accurate representations on earth. Even out of our good desire to serve God, like Aaron in Exodus 32, we craft our own versions of the golden calf in an attempt to contain an uncontainable God. Inside each one of us lives a boy who finds safety in his obedience and clarity in defined rules and regulations. Though he may also rebel against those same boundaries, something inside him rests just in knowing where they are.

Instead of judging my younger man, after significant heart work in this area, I am able to look at him with kindness, knowing he had to create God in his image in order for that same God to topple the idol and invite him to the end of himself. Indeed, if "the ability to move beyond black or white, good or evil, helpful or harmful, signals wisdom's presence,"[7] then I welcome the idol-destroying grace of God all the more. "Lay aside immaturity and live, and walk in the way of insight," wisdom calls to us in Proverbs 9:6.[8] The older we get, and the more we intentionally enter the second half of our lives, the more familiar the voice of Wisdom becomes and the less committed to either-or theologies we remain.

As a counselor, I sit with people in some of the darkest and yet most holy places of their trauma stories. The ravage of evil is far-reaching, and the extent to which darkness will go to steal, kill, and destroy the face of one of God's glorious sons or daughters is extreme. I wrestle regularly with the beauty and terror of knowing and not-knowing, holding out hope while simultaneously weeping in the ashes of people's devastation. Yes, God is God, and He is strong and loving and near. And yet, in those moments when evil showed up with its malevolence and decimation, for some reason God did not prevent it. This mystery confounds me. It always has, and it always will. But rather than lose my faith altogether or power-up and attempt to wrestle a logical answer from the doctrine books, I am invited to join the Apostle Paul as he throws up his theological hands and declares: "Oh, the depth of the riches of the wisdom and knowledge of God! How unsearchable his judgments, and his paths beyond tracing out! Who has known the mind of the Lord? Or who has been his counselor?"[9] And I settle into knowing that I simply cannot know.

As we grow and mature into our Sage, we must leave behind the either-or thinking of the first half. For those earlier years, the rules, the laws, and the checkboxes served us well, and many of us found great comfort in knowing what we thought we knew. However, "mature people are not either-or thinkers, but they bathe in the ocean of both-and."[10] On the journey towards creating a generous spirituality, we must give up our addiction to binaries and allow ourselves to *not know,* to live in the space between. This is not a move away from the good news of Jesus, but a move deeper into the mystery of God's greatness that extends beyond our human ability to comprehend. For centuries in the Church, our desert fathers and mothers have beckoned us toward the unknown and hidden mysteries of God. These Christian mystics[11] help us create the expansive faith that is a benchmark of a man in his second half.

The ancient civilizations inhabiting these rugged islands of Ireland and England knew something of this in-between space. The most holy moments of the day stood at dawn and dusk, times they called the "time between times" or "thin spaces." They also experienced certain places of worship as "thin," where the veil between this world and the next seemed semi-transparent and misty rather than shut off or closed. It is the same paradox Jesus invites us to inhabit as he reveals to us the kingdom come and the kingdom *yet* to come. Mystery, we learn, seems to be part of God's great revelation. Today we call this in-between a "liminal space," as if stepping over a threshold with one foot in and one still out. The closer a man gets to the next life, the more he recognizes the liminality of our entire existence.[12]

No more than a fifteen-minute walk from where my warm Irish cottage peat-fire currently blazes, angry waves crash against hundred-foot cliffs. As far as I can see, thick seafoam covers the surface of the water, churned over and over again by the relentless tide. Twice now I have gone to the shore to watch the tempest shoot water hundreds of feet in the air in the crash of a thunderous Irish dance. In this liminal space between earth and sea, I marvel at the co-existence of the angry violence of the waves and the stalwart unyielding grace of the rock—one forceful, the other absorbing. It is a holy place. Though no manmade temple has been erected here, it is sacred ground, for in the very same moment and same place, the both/and exists in spectacular form. Despite the thunderous booms and the occasional spray, my soul finds rest there in the in-between. And sometimes, if the sun peeks out from behind the clouds even for a moment, I can see a rainbow promising God's nearness to us all.

Stepping through the threshold of the second passage, we must lay aside our contained theologies and organized doctrines and stretch our beliefs beyond what our first-half selves might have dared. Wisdom invites us to create within ourselves a vast landscape able to, and indeed excited to, marvel at the expansive mysteries of God. Rather than occupying our theological land like the Warriors and Kings of our first half, we join the Sages of the past as they wander and wonder with awe and delight at the ever-*un*knowingness of God.

Wisdom is not born from knowledge alone, but from extensive and spacious prayer, seasons of immense and confusing suffering, and the breaking of the inner idols we have crafted by which we once garnered spiritual control over our lives. To be a wise man, we must take up residence in the liminal space of the in-between, for it is there we actually find a God who is both near yet far, loving yet angry, present yet absent, human yet God. The wisdom of the second half takes us down pathways our younger self considered too dark or too dangerous. But "if we could let go of our own obsession with what we think is the meaning of it all, we might be able to hear His call and follow Him in His mysterious, cosmic dance....we are invited to forget ourselves on purpose, [and] cast our awful solemnity to the winds."[13]

More than believe in him, God wants us to dance with him.

Much more could be said about the downward journey of second-half spirituality, but I leave that to those wise and mature men and women further down the road than I have yet traveled. Their insight, wisdom, and invitation inspire me to grow even more as a Sage. There is far more for me to explore, far more for me to unlearn and unknow. So again, I join Paul in his quest to descend into the fullness of knowing Christ: "Not that I have already obtained all this, or have already arrived at my goal, but I press on to take hold of that for which Christ Jesus took hold of me."[14]

In addition to the Sage's settled contentedness, his inner spacious hospitality, and his participation in the theological dance of unknowing, resulting in a generous spirituality, he is also a man painfully familiar with the dark valleys of suffering and grief. For him to offer hope to the world around him, he must first enter the tomb through the crucible of suffering.

QUESTIONS TO CONSIDER AND DISCUSS:

- *What has been your theological journey?*
- *In what ways have you come to the end of your theological rope? Where do you wrestle with doubt, confusion, and the "not knowing"?*
- *How do you engage with mystery, particularly as it pertains to God and faith?*
- *When considering this sort of generous spirituality, what fears do you have? What do you lose? What do you gain?*
- *Into what "unknowing" do you sense God inviting you?*

13
THE SAGE'S DEATH: THE CRUCIBLE OF SUFFERING

On April 18, 2007, my coworker Mike abruptly entered the room with a look of urgency not typical for his jovial New Zealander demeanor. I sat next to a national staff[1] friend, translating his testimony into English for the visiting American church group gathered around us. The haze of morning still covered the city, and the smell of coal fires hung heavy in the air. The day had just begun, and I could not imagine what might have caused such turmoil in Mike. Quickly excusing myself from the room, I followed him down the hall to where we could speak privately.

Mike served in multiple roles on the national leadership team for our missions organization, including taking responsibility for emergency preparedness. Over the previous months, he had received training to assist our team in the event of natural disaster, as earthquakes commonly shook our country, or in political turmoil, as we served in the ever-volatile Middle East during the years right after 9/11. But nothing could prepare Mike for this.

"Something has happened in our other office," he said. "I don't know what it is yet, but something terrible has happened."

Over the course of the next several hours, we put together puzzle pieces of information coming from our on-the-ground staff, national news agencies, our local friends, and U.S. Embassy contacts. We could not believe the horror of the truth: a band of five young men pretending to be interested in hearing about Jesus in order to gain access to our office viciously murdered three of our colleagues in a bloody massacre. Locking the door to our agency's office behind them, they bound, gagged, and tortured our friends Necati, Tillman and Ugur, killing them ritualistically in a manner meant to desecrate their bodies and make a public statement about Christian missionary activity in the country. Miraculously, local police captured these young men as they attempted to flee the scene, blood still on their hands and rage still in their hearts.

Despite their immediate arrest, fear ricocheted through our entire staff team. As one of the five members of our organization's national leadership team, with two of them outside the country and one of them now dead, it fell to me and one other national to manage and lead through the crisis. In the moments and days following the attack, we still knew very little, including the nature or the extent of their plan. Were our other offices in danger? Should we go into lockdown? Leave the country? What about our national staff? The world now looked our way, as CNN, BBC, and CBN picked up the story. Our undercover missionary operations now made national and international news, all while we attempted to tend to the crisis at hand.

Two of the deceased had families, and the third left behind a fiancée. Our agency's office in that city, from which we deployed our Bible distribution and correspondence projects, became a crime scene, and police now had unhindered access to our files, computers, and contacts. On paper, I was part-owner of the publishing company, and local papers printed my name in association with the situation. Our missionary work now exposed, news agencies smelled blood in the water, swarming us with phone calls and stationing paparazzi outside our homes. I had to use all of my 6'3" frame to fend off reporters as I escorted the widows, children, and coffins from the airport to the cemetery for the funeral.

Throughout the weeks that followed, we had very little time for grief. Unexpected waves of anguish crashed over me, reducing me to tears on the floor of the bathroom. As our crisis team made decision after decision, we often found ourselves weeping in each other's arms, barely able to hold back the crushing sorrow. Not only did we have a current emergency to manage, we had lost our dear friends in one of the most horrific ways possible.

Two weeks before he was murdered, I shared a hotel room at a conference with Necati. In between sessions he rushed back to the room to work on a paper for his seminary class, the last step to becoming a pastor. Gentle, kind, and intelligent, he embodied the grace of the gospel. On the day we parted ways from the hotel, he said to me, "Let's share a room again next time. You slept like a lamb." Those were the last words I ever heard him say.

I was 34 years old at the time of the murders. And while I had journeyed through seasons of intense suffering before, none compared to this. The moment Mike interrupted my meeting and walked me down the hall, I had no idea I was entering a season of suffering like none other. Now, 15 years later, these moments remain just as vivid in my memory as when they first occurred. Trauma does that. It digs deep ruts in our neuropathways and locks painful moments into our psyches. The ability to navigate grief is not a skill most first-half men possess, but it is vital for the Sage to learn.

VALLEYS OF DEATH

Nothing can prepare us for suffering, yet we must live with the awareness and sobriety that such suffering is part of every man's experience. No one wants it, and I have yet to meet a man who would ever willingly return to it. Grief and suffering are, however, a crucible for the soul, where the white-hot flames of pain and sorrow transform a man's heart, fundamentally moving him forward in life's journey. Lamenting the struggle that has befallen him, Frodo shares with Gandalf his wish for a different path. Wisely, Gandalf responds, "So do I, and so do all who live to see such times. But that is not for them to decide. All we have to decide is what to do with the time that is given us."[2] Suffering is a necessary part of a man's life, for it proves his heart like a crucible proves metal, purifying it and melting it so that it can be recast and remade into a new mold, the mold of a second-half Sage.

The writers of the New Testament have much to say about suffering. They readily recognize its importance and frequently invite their followers to turn towards it rather than away. In Romans, the Apostle Paul provides us with a clear pathway of suffering. He says, "We also glory in our sufferings, because we know that suffering produces perseverance; perseverance, character; and character, hope. And hope does not put us to shame."[3] According to Paul, suffering *produces*. It generates something new in us, a perseverance that then generates character, which in turn generates hope. When a man enters the dark caves of suffering, the man is transformed into a hope-filled beacon of light.

You see, suffering leaves its mark on a man. Those who have allowed suffering to shape them have an air about them, a calming presence that speaks hope despite the growing darkness around them. They see beyond the current moment because they have traversed this dark territory before and come out the other side. They believe that "[i]f we are courageous enough, care enough about our lives, we may, through suffering, get our lives back."[4] They know how to enter the valley of death and yet not fear the evil residing there. These men have fought for their lives in the pits of hell and won.

Likewise, James, the man who witnessed the gruesome crucifixion and death of his brother, Jesus, admonishes us to welcome suffering with joy as a road to maturity. He says, "Consider it pure joy, my brothers and sisters, whenever you face trials of many kinds, because you know that the testing of your faith produces perseverance. Let perseverance finish its work so that you may be *mature and complete*, not lacking anything."⁵

For those of us who long to grow into the mature Sages God designed and the world needs, the pathway is through the crucible of suffering. There is no other way.

Three general possibilities exist for how a man navigates the dark seasons of suffering: in denial, in contempt, or in reflective acceptance. Only one transforms a man into a Sage.

DENIAL: IT'S REALLY NOT THAT BAD

He left a voicemail, asking me to call when I had a chance. Lance's voice sounded calm and normal, as if his question involved something as menial as scheduling an oil change. Knowing what he and his family had recently walked through, his nonchalant message raised significant red flags, and I quickly and warily returned his call.

"Hey, Chris," he said. "I'm just calling to make sure we have all of our billing taken care of. Just buttoning some things up on my end."

"Yes, Lance," I responded, with curiosity in my voice. "Everything is clear with your account, and it looks like all the counseling sessions for you and your family have been paid. Nothing is left outstanding that I can see...*and how are you*? I haven't heard from you in a while despite trying several times to reach you."

"Oh, yeah, sorry. Things have been busy, but we are good," came his brief reply.

"Lance, that's good to hear, I think. I'm sure you have had a lot to manage these past few months." I carefully weighed my words, saying, "And these have not been months any father would want to walk through. I can imagine you've been holding a lot."

"Yeah, sure. It's been tough. But God is good, and he knows what he's doing. I'm sure there is a purpose in all of this. I'm just waiting for him to show me," he said coldly, blowing off my curiosity and care. "Anyway, thanks for letting me know our accounts are clear. Talk to you later!" And with that, he hung up the phone.

I sat back in my chair, heartbroken for Lance and his family. The reality is, three months before this call, Lance's 17-year-old son took his life by driving off the edge of a cliff. In a very public "f-you!" to his parents, he ended what had been a tumultuous and painful relationship with them by taking matters into his own hands. The young man had been in counseling, though only sporadically because Lance refused to have anyone else besides him speak into his son's life. Now, no one could speak to him at all.

The death of a child, not to mention losing one to suicide, is among the greatest tragedies a father can face. Having walked with several parents through this horrific loss, I have witnessed how incredibly crushing the avalanche of grief can be. And indeed, should be. Yet this conversation with Lance evidenced the posture of his heart–closed off, turned away, and in firm denial of the agony he simply could not face. As a result, he went about life as normal, taking care of things, crossing to-do's off his list, and organizing his external world as a way to negate his internal terror. I got to experience first-hand the denying father his now deceased son tried to warn the world about. It was heartbreaking.

We all know where this is headed for such men. The unaddressed agony will build within him a subterranean time bomb that only a volcanic eruption will dissipate. Lance will careen toward an explosive end, where he will have a mental, emotional, relational, or physical breakdown. In truth, he is on the road to losing his remaining children, divorcing his wife, or meeting an E.R. cardiologist. Those are his options.

> **Unless suffering is met and engaged, where truth is given its full weight and we acknowledge the crushing horror of grief with our full face, we will not emerge again.**

Unless suffering is met and engaged, where truth is given its full weight and we acknowledge the crushing horror of grief with our full face, we will not emerge again. Until Lance takes the bold and necessary steps toward his suffering rather than away from it, he will never be able to enter his second half. Lance will never become a Sage without entering and engaging his suffering.

CONTEMPT: SOMEONE HAS TO PAY

They started seeing me for marriage counseling during my internship in Seattle after four other therapists failed to "fix" their relationship. Several months prior, Shawn discovered Courtney's secret addiction to pornography,[6] one that had been present the entire seven years of their marriage. He was simultaneously enraged and devastated and promptly kicked her out of the house, demanding she seek personal help. Drawing a firm line, he told her, "You fix this, or you will never see your children again."

Repentant and obedient, Courtney pursued several of the porn-recovery programs in the Seattle area, a city full of resources for those caught in the dark web of the sex industry. She attended Sexaholics Anonymous (SA) meetings, read multiple books, signed up for every form of accountability software, and confessed to her friends, parents, and pastor. She pursued personal counseling with several of the published "experts,"[7] and she even went to a three-month detox program in New York for a firm reset of her life and soul. Courtney followed Shawn's demands precisely and did everything possible to redeem and restore their relationship. She, too, was devastated by what her addiction had cost them both.

Despite all her efforts and the total elimination of pornography from her life, it was never enough for Shawn. Their previous unhelpful counselor told Shawn that Courtney still evidenced an unrepentant heart because she "didn't serve him enough" and "thought too highly of herself," increasing his rage toward her and deepening his inability to move towards healing and reconciliation. They sat on my couch in one final desperate plea for help before he served the divorce papers he had already drawn up. As a leader in their church, he simply could not be married to an "unrepentant" woman, and he had already gathered support from their congregation to ex-communicate her and stand by his side.

But despite my efforts to help them unlearn the counsel they had previously received, Shawn could not move away from the contempt that had rooted in his heart. He felt it was his right to rage at Courtney's betrayal, to forever make her pay for what she did and how she made him feel. His shame over the situation blinded him with anger, and he refused to allow Jesus to heal his heart or their love. They eventually divorced, and within a year he re-married. His new wife, however, regularly met the sharp edge of his resentment and felt him sinking into a black hole of depression. The tentacles of contempt do not easily release a heart.

When we step past our denial, we often find ourselves in a place of anger. How could this be? Why me? What did I do to deserve this? How could he/she/they do this to me? Shortly after rage comes resentment, followed by depression and despair, and finally contempt. I am sure you know several men who are what we've come to name "grumpy old men." Nothing is right, good, or helpful. No one can do enough to alleviate their suffering. They have taken up residence with the curtains of their heart drawn and refuse to allow suffering to lead toward maturity. Or possibly, they have taken their rage to the office, skyrocketing up the corporate ladder while leaving carnage and debris in their wake. They find in their contempt a fuel for their lives, seeking revenge but never finding relief. Like all of us, they have faced seasons of suffering in their lives, but instead of moving *through* the anger, they found comfort and power in it, feeding their hatred and giving them sufficient reason to avoid the vulnerability of love again. Men like this take their pain and turn it back on the world. Someone has to pay.

REFLECTIVE ACCEPTANCE: PAIN BECOMES LOVE

And then, there are those men who recognize suffering not only for what it takes from us, but also for what it gives us. As I have said, no one willingly invites a season of pain. But when those inevitable moments come, these men turn *towards* it, lean into it, and give themselves over to the gift of grief.

I grew up knowing one such man. His name was Leonard. Born in the early 1900s as the last of eight children, Leonard was the son of the parish pastor in a small farming town in rural Oklahoma. Leo grew up all boy, with scraped knees, a perpetually dirty face, and a deep love for animals. He did his chores and succeeded at his studies, earning him a position in medical school on the other side of the state. At the age of 24, he graduated as a doctor and started his career in medicine after meeting his wife at a local dance. Though they struggled with infertility at first, their miracle baby was born after five years of trying, and then they tried again for another nine years before baby number two came along.

A few years later Leo noticed his wife's increasing struggle to catch her breath as she tended to the children. Over the course of a few months and several tests, it became clear she had developed a slow-growing, yet untreatable, form of lung cancer. For several years, she fought valiantly with moments of remission offering her precious time with her husband and children. But ultimately, Leo's wife succumbed to the disease when her youngest was 14 years old.

Leo, then a 45-year-old single parent and widower in the 1950s, grieved long and deep. He had lost his love, along with all their hopes and dreams and wild plans to move to the Alaskan frontier to provide medical services to the underserved Alaskan natives. It all came to a screeching halt with her passing. At times, it seemed too much to bear, and his children often heard him crying in bed at night.

After what felt like a lengthy season, though the grief did not end, it lessened enough for him to continue working as a doctor in Oklahoma. He never remarried, choosing instead to devote himself to his children and then, eventually, to his grandchildren. For the next 45 years, he focused his mind and heart on bringing the love of God to his family, always being the "fun" grandparent, the one who cared little for what was proper and more for what brought joy and delight. When his grown children needed him, he was there, not offering advice unless asked, but instead providing enough space for their grief to live, be attended to, and grow them as well. He died at age 94, having lived a life of meaning and creating a legacy. Though marred by many other seasons of suffering, he always faced forward, knowing the only way out of suffering is through it.

In his excellent book *Turn My Mourning into Dancing: Finding Hope in Hard Times,* Nouwen invites us to engage suffering this same way. He writes,

> Instead, Christ invites us to remain in touch with the many sufferings of every day and to taste the beginning of hope and new life right there, where we live amid our hurts and pains and brokenness....I am less likely to deny my suffering when I learn how God uses it to mold me and draw me closer to him. I will be less likely to see my pains as interruptions to my plans and more able to see them as the means for God to make me ready to receive him. I let Christ live near my hurts and distractions.[8]

Every Sage I have ever known has walked dark roads of suffering. The crucible of pain and grief are familiar to him, and he lives with a proven and sober knowledge of its refining yet restorative heat. In fact, no man can enter the second half and step fully into the role of Sage until he has followed the path of Jesus: into death, through hell, and back again.

The word "patience" originates from the Latin word *patior*, meaning "to suffer." As we grow into second-half men, our patience increases as we learn to suffer hardship rather than deny it or rage against it. One great hallmark of a Sage is his unnerving patience, his willingness to wait, endure, and observe the unfolding story. First-half men are often in a great hurry, worried about losing opportunities or making deadlines. Sages do not honk horns or demand others get out of the way; instead, they suffer the delay and anticipate their arrival in due time. Again, Nouwen wisely tells us, "For in our suffering, not apart from it, Jesus enters our sadness, takes us by the hand, pulls us gently up to stand, and invites us to dance."[9] It is through our suffering, not despite it, we learn a deeper gladness not connected to our circumstances, successes, or comforts.

After the horrendous murders of my friends, I entered a three-year season of confusion, mourning, and grief. One year prior to that awful day, my wife and I had decided to return to the United States to attend seminary in order to retool and retrain for the next season of ministry. April 18, 2007, came just six weeks before our scheduled departure, and it was in those last days of a decade-long career as an international missionary—a time that should be full of sweet remembrances and celebratory goodbyes—that I faced the most horrendous moment of my leadership career. Upon arrival at grad school in Seattle, Beth and I knew no one and found ourselves shell-shocked and grateful for the simplicity of wooded parks, open spaces, and a Trader Joe's around the corner.

As a counseling student, I was fortunate to have professors and fellow students who were aware and attuned enough to see I was truly not well. Kindly and deftly, they cared for my grieving heart, welcoming the torrents of my emotions with the tenderness of Jesus. I thought no one would understand what I felt since murder and martyrdom were not a common experience in the American church. It took two years for Beth and I to emerge from grief enough to tell our newly found Seattle friends about the tragedy we endured just before our arrival. And slowly, I found my feet again, able to offer others the generous spaciousness of sorrow I had visited for so long. While I would never wish this experience upon anyone, I am grateful to have walked through seasons of suffering such as this for the refinement the fire has brought me.

Even one of my favorite fictional Sages, Gandalf the Gray, faces his greatest trial when he squares off and sacrifices himself to the fiery Balrog in the Mines of Moria in order to save his friends. Through trial, pain, suffering, and death, he returns to Middle Earth as an even greater Sage, Gandalf the White. It is true: "Authentic suffering requires encounters with dragons."[10] No one is exempt from the crucible of suffering, and the more we become familiar with those dark paths, the more we find space for the light of Jesus.

Engaging our suffering through grief transforms our wounds from festering to victorious. The very wounds responsible for the death of Jesus, those in his hands and side, became for many the good news and proof of life after death. Through resurrection, those wounds transformed into beacons of hope for those who followed him. His disciple Thomas wisely demanded to see and touch Jesus's wounds, knowing that healed wounds point to suffering that has been redeemed. What was once broken, bruised, and torn is now healed. Not removed. Not gone. Not disappeared. But healed. *This* is the hope of the victorious Christ.

Living inside every man is a boy who knows pain, sorrow, suffering, and grief. Rather than deny the wounding or rage against it, we must acknowledge the depth of our losses, mourn with our own younger parts for what they have suffered, and tend to the broken hearts longing to taste the salt of another's tears. To acknowledge his suffering is not to admit weakness but strength. That boy has suffered much and survived. For us to step through the second passage and into the Sage, we must suffer and suffer well, for suffering produces maturity and wisdom. Without healed wounds of his own, a Sage cannot walk wisely or hopefully with a suffering world.

As we continue our exploration into the six distinctive qualities of a Sage, let's recall our journey thus far: we started with a settled contentedness, leading the way to spacious inner hospitality and a generous spirituality. The deep valleys of suffering transform a man's hope and free his heart to be anchored in a home not yet realized. Additionally, a true Sage must learn the secret of solitude over loneliness, becoming friends with himself and discovering there a renewal of God's masterful design.

QUESTIONS TO CONSIDER AND DISCUSS:

- *How was suffering engaged in your childhood home? Was it?*
- *In the face of suffering, if you were to tend towards denial or contempt, which would it be? Why?*
- *What would you identify as your life's most significant seasons of suffering? What happened, and how did you navigate those dark valleys?*
- *What does it mean to you to "suffer well?" How might suffering be generative?*
- *What suffering remains untended in your life? What would you like to do with that now?*

14

THE SAGE'S COMPANION: FROM LONELINESS TO SOLITUDE

Today I wake to the sound of wind and rain swirling forcefully around my Irish cottage. Built more than 50 years ago of cinder block and mortar, I am sure this structure has endured far worse. In fact, it does not even shudder despite the tempest outside. The windows titter with the rain, and the wind echoes down the chimney. Though I quickly build a fire to take the chill out of the morning air, I doubt it will do much to battle the elements. Still, the licking and dancing flames, the crackle of the wood, and the smell of burning Irish peat bring comfort and companionship on this dark morning.

The sun does not rise until late morning, usually around 8:30 a.m. or so, though the surrounding hills keep the village in shadow until almost 10. There are no streetlights on these small single-lane roads, and one must carry a light to see at night as the clouds so often hide the moon and stars. The sun disappears before 5 p.m. This can be a dark and lonesome place.

Yesterday, in an effort to "get out," I took the local shuttle, trading my village (population 159) for the bustle of the neighboring town (population 2,050).[1] There, I shopped for groceries, went to the bank, dropped my empty jars and bottles in the recycling bins near the harbor, and found some tea and lunch at the 350-year-old Benner's Hotel. I found it refreshing to get out, leave my desk and writing routine, and experience human contact once again. Though everyone there was a stranger, to see their faces and hear the lilt of their Irish brought a smile to my face.

On my way home, the shuttle picked up two older men—the same two who rode with me into town this morning. They greeted one another by name but sat apart, silently looking out the window for the entire 40 minute ride. Scruffy and weathered, they have evidently spent their lives working these farms and hills, their families having likely lived here for generations. All three of us disembarked at the final stop, and the two of them walked separately into the pub, the only establishment for miles. I have seen them there each time I have stopped in for a pint after a hike, and I have observed them. Guinness in hand, they sit at separate tables in the same vicinity. There are no words shared, or at least very few, and they stare into their glasses with vacant eyes and no sense of togetherness. The only camaraderie is in the communal experience of isolation and loneliness.

THE LONELINESS CRISIS

The Center for Disease Control and Prevention (CDC) has identified loneliness, especially for older men, as a significant contributor to serious health conditions.[2] Multiple studies show a staggering number of older adults at increased risk of several mental and physical health concerns due to loneliness and social isolation. This was true even prior to the COVID-19 pandemic, which only exponentially increased the social separation between people, especially the vulnerable older population. In fact, both Japan and the United Kingdom implemented a new Minister of Loneliness after an alarming increase in suicide and other life-threatening health-related concerns were tied to loneliness.[3] Despite the rapid increase of technologies designed to connect the world and extend our lives, loneliness remains one of the leading factors of health decline for those over age 50. As a result, loneliness has been deemed its own epidemic.[4]

When I initially shared my plan to head to Ireland for a secluded month of reflection, prayer, and writing, almost without fail, the first question people asked was, "Won't you be lonely?" or "Is Beth going with you?" When I answered, "No, and she's actually blessing me and *sending* me," the immediate retort was, "Not even for a visit?!" No, not even for a visit.

Indeed, I am among the many who consider themselves introverts, those who recharge internally by getting space and time alone. While I enjoy being with people, getting to know their stories, engaging in conversation, and participating in play, co-creation, and dialogue, I am refreshed and renewed when I can retreat into my own head and heart to process the world around me. But it is not introversion that called me to this place, nor is it what makes being here bearable for these dark January days. Rather, it is the invitation to the practice of solitude, a spiritual discipline every Sage must master. And while not every man has the opportunity to retreat to a place such as this to grow his capacity for solitude, every man must find ways in his own life, right where he is, to pursue it. Solitude, in fact, is a choice.

THE GUYS

Many men remember with great fondness the friendships they had with other guys in high school, college, or the military. The bonds were deep, and the brotherhood formed during those years was intimate, personal, life-changing, and powerful. As my son finishes his senior year of college, he is always with "the guys." Even though many of them are dating or engaged, "the guys" is a unit, a pack, a posse, and they walk through the world and everything in it *together*.

However, once the close quarters of those college years are over, and jobs and marriages and children increasingly capture their attention, the intensity of brotherhood wanes. Most men I talk with in their 30s and 40s still have a group of men they consider their "closest friends," though they only see them once or twice a year at a poker weekend or ski retreat and scarcely talk with them in between. By his 50s, if a man has not been intentional about his pursuit of masculine relationships, he will look around and find himself alone in the world.[5]

Many men tell me, "My wife is my best friend. I'd love to have other friends, but I simply don't have time or interest. She's it. Anyway, what am I supposed to do? Where am I supposed to find friends? Is there an app for guys like me?" Most happily married men know the deep goodness their wives bring to their lives. To have a partner with whom you can talk, play, explore, worship, and love is a genuine gift. But the fact is, she cannot be her husband's best friend. Just as there is something beautiful in the gathering of women, so too a unique and powerful space is created when men gather with other men. The rawness, relatability, mutual identification, and respect open parts of our lives and hearts that remain otherwise closed off and often inaccessible. To say a man needs no friend other than his wife is to put her in an unfair position to be the brother he actually needs. She needs other women. He needs other men. She needs his brothers to tend to his masculine heart so she is free to be his wife and lover, not his buddy.

Far too many men, however, spend much of their lives lonely. They do not have this brotherhood of men, and they feel hopeless to find it. Once their high school and college friendships wane, they secretly resolve to live an isolated and lonely life. The typical manhood script works against them, making vulnerability with other men unmasculine, stealing away their time and focus from cultivating friendships towards climbing ladders, and destroying true brotherhood with false teachings on man-to-man accountability.[6] The work of building adult male friendships seems too daunting, and the options feel too sparse. And yet, it is imperative for the first-half man to develop deep and lasting relationships with other men. Without them, he will increasingly lose himself and be woefully unprepared for the challenges he will face during the Zealous Warrior, Wounded Man, and Restored King stages of his life. A man without brothers will inevitably remain stuck somewhere in his masculine journey, and he cannot free himself. He needs the leveraging power of other men to dislodge him from the quagmire, show up for his family when he is taken out, and kindly, yet directly, wake him up when his second story consumes him. While it is true no one can do his internal work for him, he needs a company of men to put their hands on his back in solid and caring support through the highs and lows of life.

For this reason, one of the core initiatives of Restoration Project is brotherhood.[7] We believe men become true men through their sharpening relationships with other men, and it is in the context of brotherhood that men are most seen, known, and cared for throughout life. Men are better fathers, husbands, employers, employees, contributors to church and community, and followers of Jesus when they have an intentional cadre of men with whom they journey through life. This does not come easy, and it requires pursuit, vulnerability, time, and investment. If a man is married, it also requires his wife's blessing and buy-in, knowing he is challenged, encouraged, and cared for by other men. We all need men at our table, a collection of fellow journeymen with whom we can ally in this masculine life.

One evening during our Scotland trek five years ago, the four of us sat at a corner table in a mostly empty pub on the far reaches of the north-western coast. A fire danced in the large stone hearth, and whiskey glasses donned the table in celebration and camaraderie. Bart, Greg, Shae, and I had just completed another day of Scottish adventure, and now, as was our custom and design for this trip, we sat discussing aspects of a man's journey. Though we form our own little circle, we each live in different places and have other significant men in our lives. In the conversation about the high value of masculine friendships, the question was posed: "Who are the kings at your table?" Every man needs other kings at his table, other men who bring the fullness of their domains to bear on behalf of one another's good. The importance of this for *every* man cannot be overstated, and it is vital to form a brotherhood with intention in the first half.

FIRST-HALF LONELINESS

On this wintery Irish morning I am taking a short walk to the pier located about a half-mile from where I am staying. I pause not only to stretch my legs, but to ponder the lonely seasons of my own life. As I descend the steep and windy path down the cliffs to the landing-stage below, I find a perch halfway down, just close enough to the edge to put a lump in my throat, but low enough to escape the winds howling overhead. I have taken with me some stale bread to throw to the seagulls, and though I attempt to taunt them with an easy meal, they remain unphased and uninterested in my presence. Those words jar my thoughts...unphased and uninterested.

I am reminded of a moment early on in the Warrior stage of my life. Having arrived for our first year-long stint overseas, my wife and I served on a small team with one other American couple, two national interns, and a national staff as our leader. The year proved exceedingly difficult as we navigated a challenging language barrier, tension amongst the team, and eventually ethically questionable actions by one of our overseers. Toward the halfway mark of that year, as I rode public transportation alone to share the gospel on a college campus, I thought to myself, "No one knows what is going on for me. No one knows how I am, what I'm doing, or what I feel. The only other American man on this team doesn't know. The only person remotely close to knowing is Beth. Thank God for her. But everyone else is unphased and uninterested in my presence." I felt impotent in my work, unknown by my leadership, and lonely in a foreign land without a single man to call "friend."

Later that week, I gathered the courage to talk to my American teammate, lamenting with him how lonely it all was. Not surprisingly, he felt similar. And while we made significant headway towards a deeper relationship, he and his wife finished the year and moved back to the States. Since that experience, I have resolved to intentionally pursue men, to find a cadre of guys to sit together as kings at the table, fighting, grieving, ruling, building, and becoming men together. It has been an incredible journey, and together with these brothers, I have been shaped and chiseled and rescued in my first half.

A man who is lonely in his first half will continue to be lonely well into his older years, and therefore, the likelihood of true brotherhood at this stage decreases. Old men generally do not make new friends. They may find a golfing or travel buddy, but the ache of loneliness has already taken root. The Irish men down the street from me now, sitting at Krugers Pub and staring at the bottom of yet another empty pint of Guinness, may be in each other's presence, and may have even known each other for decades, yet it is painfully evident to even the most cursory of observers, there is no brotherhood there. They are lonely old men who will come back tomorrow for another round.

For a man to cross through the second passage into Sage, he must take all he has gained from the brotherhood of his first half and learn yet a new lesson, the lesson of

Loneliness and solitude do not coexist.

solitude. The awareness, the care, the containment, and the blessing he received from his brothers now provide him with the firm internal foundation on which he stands as a second-half man. As he has learned to be vulnerable with other men, he now has the capacity to be vulnerable with himself. As he has discovered how to be friends with others, he now has the capacity to be friends with himself. His brothers have helped him hold fast to the masterpiece of God within, and as he steps into his second half, he now takes charge of holding fast to his own masterpiece himself. Through the reflection of his brothers, he has come to love his own face. While he does not abandon his seat at the table, the wars he now fights are with his own internal dragons in the realm where no other man can join him, the realm of solitude. Loneliness and solitude do not coexist.

LONELINESS, ALONENESS, AND SOLITUDE

Frequently, solitude is confused with loneliness and aloneness. As we press into our understanding of solitude as a comfortable spiritual practice of a Sage, we must first clearly define what it is and what it is not. Of the three—solitude, loneliness, and aloneness—only solitude is considered an ancient Christian "spiritual practice," receiving significant attention from many church mothers and fathers across time, including John the Baptist, the family of Basil the Great (whose sons helped author the Nicene Creed and whose daughters led monastic communities), St. Francis of Assisi, Thomas Merton, and Father Richard Rohr. Throughout history, those whom we now consider "Sages of the church" regularly retreated from the world to find themselves and God through the practice of solitude. To this day, monasteries, abbeys, hermitages, and contemplative retreat centers offer opportunities for modern-day believers to exercise solitude.

Nouwen provides an excellent summary of the differences between loneliness, aloneness, and solitude:

> Solitude, to begin, does not mean so much withdrawing in silence out of antisocial sentiments. Solitude means that our aloneness sometimes does not come as a sad fact needing healing but rather offers a place where God comes to bring communion. In fact, solitude has rich roots and connotations significantly different from two other words often associated with it: *Aloneness* generally means being by oneself in a neutral way. *Loneliness* more suggests the pain of desolation or another's absence. But solitude carries notes of joy and possibility. For solitude, for the Christian, means

not just to wander off to the woods or desert or mountaintop for private withdrawal. It means daring to stand in God's presence. Not to guard time simply to be alone, but alone in God's company.[8]

There is great purpose in solitude, for solitude involves pursuit as well as withdrawal. It is not merely isolating oneself from others, but doing so in order to silence the noise and distraction that keeps us from encountering God and our own selves. It is in this space a man finds the face and companionship of God. The Sage moves from settled contentedness to inner hospitality, and then embraces a generous spirituality, which allows him the freedom and hope of meeting himself and God in the space of quiet solitude.

When Moses returned from his 40 days of solitude on Mt. Sinai, Exodus 34:29 tells us, "he was not aware that his face was radiant because he had spoken with the Lord."[9] The glory of God had been revealed to Moses, and it lingered on his face for all to see. Per the request of the Israelites, he covered his face *until* he again entered the presence of God. When he was there in that solitary place, Moses removed the veil to speak with God face to face. And each time, the radiance of God shone.[10] The scripture teems with examples of sagely solitude. Consider Jesus and his 40 days of solitude in the wilderness, wrestling against the wiles of the enemy for the establishment of the true kingdom on earth. Or the Apostle John exiled on the island of Patmos as he encountered the revelatory Christ and received the words recorded in the Book of Revelation. Or the dreamer Joseph and his years of isolation in prison. Or Elijah. Or Paul. Spend time with any man you consider a "Sage," a man whose face exudes the kindness and love of God, and you will find he is friends with solitude.

Partnered with solitude is the practice of silence. We live in a world of distraction, where everyone in the known universe has unhindered access to your time and attention. Phones, watches, computers, tablets, smart cars, and smart-home devices (to name but a few) buzz and ding and notify you constantly of what you should immediately consider is of utmost importance. We fill our ears with news, podcasts, music, and audio books, and we barrage our eyes with never-ending screens. Despite my currently remote Irish hermitage, I count four screens within five feet of where I sit: my computer, iPad, phone, and the TV that hangs on the wall. Equally challenging to practice as solitude, silence requires a focused and intentional unplugging and retreat. Of the importance of silence, Thomas Merton said:

> This then is what it means to seek God perfectly: to withdraw from illusion and pleasure, from worldly anxieties and desires…to keep my mind free from confusion in order that my liberty may be always at the disposal of His will; to entertain silence in my heart and listen for the voice of God…to gather all that I am, and have all that I can possibly suffer or do or be, and abandon them all to God in the resignation of perfect love….*Bonum est praestolari cum silentio salutare Dei.* (It is good to wait in silence for the salvation of God.)[11]

Silence makes space for the heart to hear the voice of God. Solitude without silence is like rain without water. The two are inseparable. For us to know and experience the whispering presence of God, we must cease, desist, and quiet our minds and spirits. As the Psalmist tells us, "For God alone my soul waits in silence, for my hope is from him."[12] To be silent is to humble ourselves before the presence of God, waiting for him to speak and opening our hearts to listen. It is, as Merton said, gathering all of who we are, all the parts of our lives and stories, all the lost, broken, exiled, and scared younger parts who live within us, to bring them to the solitary place where God meets us with his love. Silence and solitude invite us to become friends with ourselves as we are befriended by God.

> Together with silence, solitude transforms a man from the god of his own world into a Sage for the High King.

Inside every man is a lonely boy who needs *someone* to be his friend, and it is here he is not only found, but welcomed and enjoyed.

Together with silence, solitude transforms a man from the god of his own world into a Sage for the High King.

Loneliness, on the other hand, is borne from the pain of our disappointed projections. When we rely on those in our external world to bring validation, purpose, meaning, and identity to fill the chasm of our aching unmet needs, loneliness becomes a consuming fire. They can never be all we need them to be, and no matter how much they offer, it will never be enough. But when we transform our loneliness into an encounter with ourselves, becoming friends with our own divine masterpiece in partnership with the One who created us in the first place, we come face to face with God. It is no accident that all ancient church fathers and mothers, as well as the modern-day fictional Sages to which I often refer (i.e. Yoda and Dumbledore), have secret hideaways in distant places, secluded from the world in order to discover the soul-transforming gift of solitude.

To pass over the threshold of the second half, a man must become well-acquainted with solitude. If he is to survive this second passage, he must face the ache of loneliness to achieve oneness with himself and God. Learning solitude is a prerequisite to becoming a Sage.

Jesus also knew these secret places, finding regular refuge in the wilderness while in the presence of his Father. It is no surprise that

> The clarity of thought and action that would later characterize Jesus' public ministry came from his years of preparation in solitude and anonymity. The core of that preparation was meeting God in the secret place of his inner self. It was through meeting God in places of solitude that Jesus discovered his identity and grew in intimacy with God.[13]

As we become more like Christ, growing up into maturity, transforming into the Sages God has designed us to be, how much more should we pursue the gift of solitude?

"But who will you talk to? What will you do? That much solitude would kill me," I frequently heard before boarding the plane for this month-long Irish experience of solitude.

"Myself," I replied. "I will talk to myself. We are slowly becoming good friends."

PRACTICING SOLITUDE

I am not naive to the fact that my month's journey to Ireland is a practical impossibility for most men. It has indeed been an uncommon experience. And yet, while you may not be able to plan such a trip in your pursuit of solitude, I invite you to consider just how you might create the time and space to take intentional steps toward it. Several people have told me, "Well, I can't do *that*, so I guess I'll settle for a quiet Sunday afternoon."

In this statement, I hear two things. First, a thousand yeses to the quiet sabbath. When you have the opportunity to take space for solitude, take it in whatever form it may come. Whether it is a few hours or a few days, it will require purposed intention, along with agreement and assistance from others in your life, to create moments of solitude. They simply do not happen on their own. Even if a man has an "afternoon free," he often fills it with chores, watching sports, or other dutiful activities. My recommendation is to "take and make" opportunities for solitude. Otherwise, it will never happen.

But the second thing I hear in this statement is the fated word "settle." Far too many men settle, accepting their fate with either resignation or resentment, and give up the intentioned pursuit of their own souls. This is, in my mind, soul suicide. Rather than accept what is, let us be a generation of men who reimagine what could be. If we intend to pursue solitude, where and how might that be accomplished? What help might need to be enlisted? What teaching might need to be engaged?

For several years, in my intentional pursuit of solitude, I have taken a one- or two-night personal retreat a couple of times a year. I find a reasonable yet comfortable hotel in the city next door, load up my books, comfortable sweatpants, and ear plugs, and get 24 to 48 hours on my own. Yes, there is an expense, both financially and relationally, and my wife and I sacrifice our money and our time to make this happen. In fact, we do this for each other because we believe in the purpose and buy into the vision, knowing the person who emerges from these brief windows of solitude wears a face that glows a little more with the presence of God.

Men, to become a Sage, we must pursue solitude. We must find it, for it will not find us. Only through the trials of solitude will we be able to take the next step through the second passage.

Many excellent books have been written about the discipline of solitude by saints far more practiced than me. I have found deep wisdom and inspiration from their work, and I refer you to this incredible body of literature[14] for further exploration and study. My task here has been to orient you to the necessity of solitude as a crucial part of your onward journey as a second-half man. It stands as one of the primary requirements of the Sage, for within such practiced solitude we find those parts of us we have long forgotten, hated, ignored, and exiled. As we meet there with Jesus, we are able to experience his kindness, not only from him towards us, but from ourselves towards ourselves. The reintegration of those parts back into our being only happens when we have spent enough time away from our distractions and projections and "[s]tand at the crossroads and look; ask for the ancient paths, ask where the good way is, and walk in it, and you will find rest for your souls."[15]

QUESTIONS TO CONSIDER AND DISCUSS:

- *What do you feel when you consider extended periods of solitude? Excitement? Terror? Confusion? Something else?*
- *Do a quick review of the noise in your life. How often do you have silence?*
- *If you were to "take and make" opportunities for silence and solitude, what might that look like for you?*
- *In what ways are you lonely? How have you pursued intentional masculine relationships in your first half? Have you?*
- *What might it mean for you to befriend your own self as you are befriended by God?*

15
THE SAGE'S BOY: BRINGING HIM HOME

Shalom, shalom
The Lord is in your midst
Shalom, shalom
The Lord will fight for you
He won't let go, through fair and wind and storm
Shalom, shalom
The Lord is your midst[1]

For days now, this chorus has echoed in the background of my cottage, filling the space with an air of closeness and peace. This song, along with several cello and violin compositions, has been my soundtrack. This morning I spent two hours by the fire, watching the heat on the coals dance while it warmed my body and my heart. I need a warm companion on the journey today.

I have been reflecting on those long-ago moments of my boyhood, those times burned in my memory that were but a moment and I have had no reason to revisit since. These glimpses, snapshots of my younger self in everyday life doing everyday things, have remained unvisited and dormant for 40-plus years. The living room couch. The landscaping in the backyard. The leopard costume for Halloween. The *Green Machine* my neighbor would not let me ride. The overstuffed homemade pillow I cuddled during Saturday morning cartoons. I remember the dinnertime conversations, or lack thereof. Bath time and bedtime and the chipmunk-and-forest wallpaper of my boyhood room. Seemingly unimportant moments collect over years into a vast library of memory to form the expansive narratives of our lives. Like the thousand brushstrokes of the painter, or the chisel's thousand measured tip-taps in the hands of the sculptor, these memories and moments first form the boy and then, from out of the boy, emerges the man with the boy still inside. As Madeliene L'Engle writes,

> I am still every age that I have been. Because I was once a child, I am always a child. Because I was once a searching adolescent, given to moods and ecstasies, these are still part of me, and always will be....This does not mean that I ought to be trapped or enclosed in any of these ages...but that they are in me to be drawn on; to forget is a form of suicide; my past is part of what makes the present [person] and must not be denied or rejected or forgotten.[2]

As I step into those ancient corridors of memory, I ask my younger self how he is and what he feels. I am not asking him to tell me about his hurts, fears, secrets, or traumas. I merely wonder with him what it feels like to be him, putting myself back into those younger shoes. He is not quite sure what to do with my questions, and as little boys tend to do, he starts to talk about the impressive scars he has from his many adventures.

He shows me the line under his chin where he received seven stitches from the time when he donned the Superman cape and attempted to fly *up* the brick stairs in the garden. As I remember that moment, I touch my chin and feel the thin scar line underneath my now gray whiskers. My older self connects with my younger self, and together we smile at his audacity and courage.

He shows me his deformed toe from the time he and his sister played in the sprinklers on a hot summer day. He accidentally stepped barefoot on the metal dividing the grass from the lava rocks, almost severing this toe from his foot. I take off my sock and marvel at how crooked it is, knowing now how blisters form on that toe every time I hike more than a few miles. My adult self shakes my head at the ridiculousness of such landscaping.

He points to both knees, scraped and scarred so many times he can't remember all the stories that go with them. But the man in me now knows what it takes to clean and bandage a wound, and I inspect my mother's decades-old work, at times in awe and at times with a raised brow.

He points to his right eyelid, forever marked by the guide wire from the neighbor's tree that sliced it open while he fled a game of tag. He ran home with his hand over his eye, terrified of losing his sight. I watch the memory play on the movie screen in my mind, as he sat on the counter and Mom called the doctor from the landline in the kitchen. The young boy looked at me with shared astonishment, as the pain strangely subsided and the eyelid miraculously healed in an instant, leaving only a mascara-like line as evidence of the incident.

Then my younger self shows me the scar on my right hand. It's big and in the fleshy part of the thumb. He reminds me how the razor blade accidentally skipped off the mirror as he attempted to remove a sticker, plunging deep into the muscle. Though it should have had stitches, he cleaned that one himself and hid it, not telling his parents until that night at church, knowing they could not get mad at him for his recklessness whilst they sat together in the house of God. My older self remembers the terror and the many excuses he invented to cover his extended time in the bathroom as he bandaged it and cleaned up the blood. The father's heart in me now breaks for how unfathered he was in that moment. After stoking the fire and breathing deeply to the slow rhythm of the music, I ask my boy what he was afraid his parents would do or say. Without the need for explanation, for he knows I know, he says, "Dad's look."

A torrent of memories come flooding forth, every one a moment when he experienced the pained and disappointed look of his father coupled with the desperate plea of his mother. Together we talk about the other kind of scars, the ones no one sees, the ones he has buried and dismissed as stupid, unimportant, unreal, or unmanly to acknowledge. He tells me, "I had no one to teach me or show me. I had no one."

Shalom, shalom. The Lord is in your midst.

For the next hour, my older self visits, along with my younger self, the yet untold moments of loss, shame, guilt, dismissal, and fear from his younger years all the way into his adolescence. My adult man offers space and blessing to my boy and acknowledges both the shortcomings of his dad as well as the good, brave, and emerging man growing inside him. We talk about the burgeoning masculine energy rising from within and the desire to know his strength and power and test it against his father. I remember a scene of the two of us wrestling on the floor of the family room, a moment that should exemplify a boy-to-man connection between us. But then memory's lens widens to reveal my disabled sister also attempting to participate in the wrestle-play. My younger self shows me how he has to pretend, minimize, and moderate his pounces and pins to protect her from getting hurt, fake-falling when she touches him and conceding the imaginary fight. "I had no one," he repeats.

Suddenly, the flow of memory takes me back to the leopard Halloween costume, pointing to a photograph I have seen in my parents' scrapbooks. My younger boy stands at the front door with a despondent look on his face, plastic trick-or-treat pumpkin pail in hand. Indeed, he is dressed as a leopard, whiskers and all. Or better stated, he *has been dressed* in the leopard costume. Next to him stands his sister, five years older in age but a toddler developmentally. She is dressed as Superman, complete with a cape and a felt "S" sewn onto her chest. *She* got to be Superman that year, and for every year ever since.

"I wanted to be Superman," my younger self says with tears. "I *am* Superman. But she got whatever she wanted, and I had to be the stupid leopard so it wouldn't upset her. Or upset Mom. Or Dad. But I wanted to be Superman!" The many times he shrank or stepped aside to keep the peace in the family comes into view, like a thousand smoothed rocks on a much buffeted shore. Again, tears form in my adult man's eyes as I remember what it felt like to stand at that door year after year with *my* cape around *her* neck.

"Yes, you *are* Superman. And you have the scar to prove it," I say, rubbing my chin with a boyish smile.

Though there are other stories we visited together this morning, they remain private between my boy and me. There are more. A thousand more. While I am not unfamiliar with this younger part of me as a result of the first-half storywork I have done, he has more to say, more to reveal, and more to ask. The more time I spend listening to and blessing this boy, the more I welcome him back into myself and remember the innocent desires and the glorious masterpiece he brought to this world, the more he comes home.

As Rohr tells us, "Home is both the beginning and the end."[3] For men to move further into the second half, our younger parts must find their way back. As with every hero's journey, we return to the beginning. Throughout our masculine journey, we have sought and pursued a place of Edenic hope, a home we believed existed "out there somewhere," so we set out on a lifelong quest to discover, recover, or build it for ourselves. Little did we know the "out there" actually already existed "in here." Every great hero leaves his home only to return to it in the end. When the dragon is slain, the enemy defeated, the treasure found, the invaders routed, and the peace restored, though the journey has done its work to

> For men to move further into the second half, our younger parts must find their way back.

transform him into something more, it always brings him back to where he started. He had to leave his home to find the greater home within.

A man can only take someone else as far as he himself has gone. He must walk the long and hard road of recovering his boyhood masterpiece to truly travel the second passage. Though on the outside of every tree we only see the mature tree, a careful inspection of its cross-section reveals all its rings, telling the story of every age that tree has ever lived–years of sun, rain, drought, fire and wind. In the same way, on the outside of every man we only see the adult, but internally, in the rings of his soul, lives every age, every moment, *he* has ever experienced. Though he has grown up, the little boy and the younger man still reside within him. All they have endured–seasons of shame, trauma, denial, violence, abuse, abandonment, great love, and great loss–tell the story of the adult man he has become.

As I have said, the task of the first passage is to find the man within the boy and call him forth. The task of the second passage is to find the boy within the man and bring him home.

FACING THE SHADOW: SHAME, CONTEMPT, AND DISGUST

Throughout the trauma and tragedy of our second story, where evil's vehement assault against us rages, parts of our True Self shatter under the crushing blows of abuse, neglect, dismissal, abandonment, and betrayal. Whether the trauma is large or small, our young selves splinter off as a means of survival, and we leave them behind as we try to make it through to live to another day. In those crucial moments, we may suppress our fear, recognizing our display of weakness may result in further harm. Instead, we power up and turn away from our scared selves, burying them under layers of bravado in order to protect our fearful hearts. Or we may flee from our desire for connection and relationship, learning over time how dangerous hope and vulnerability can be. As a result, we become unemotional but protected men. Or met with the unimaginable dilemma between sexual arousal and abuse, we may spiritualize our self-denial and send our passions into realms of contempt, disgust, and sin. We find safety in security, make close friends with "recovery," and latch onto false accountability as our primary means of rescuing our souls from the dangers of desire.

At times, we send those parts, those little boys, into exile, ashamed of who they are and never wanting to see them again. At other times, we allow them to remain nearby but turn our anger towards them in burning contempt for their weakness or failure. Or we turn against them in disgust, unable to withstand their brokenness or their sin.

Whether they have been exiled by our shame, burned by our contempt, or suffered the snarl of our disgust, these parts of our True Self long to be restored and brought back to the table. Paul tells us in Romans 2:4, "the kindness of God leads you to repentance."[4] Not our shame. Not our contempt. Not our disgust. Not even our obedience. *His kindness.* As we tend to the brokenhearted boys we have so purposefully disregarded with the strong tenderness of Jesus, we reintegrate them back into our hearts and return ever closer to our True Selves. "We never get to the second half of life without major shadowboxing," Rohr says. "Your shadow [i.e. the lost boys within you] is what you refuse to see about yourself, and what you do not want others to see."[5] Retrieving these boys through the kindness of God is the primary task of the second passage. The Sage recognizes the shattering of his divine masterpiece and does the hard work to partner with Jesus to restore and reintegrate that which has been broken.

The Apostle Paul begins his first letter to Timothy, his young apprentice, with a bold and relieving proclamation: *he claims to be the greatest sinner of all time.* Consider Eugene Peterson's rendition of 1 Timothy 1:12-17:

I'm so grateful to Christ Jesus for making me adequate to do this work. He went out on a limb, you know, in trusting me with this ministry. The only credentials I brought to it were violence and witch hunts and arrogance. But I was treated mercifully because *I didn't know what I was doing*—didn't know Who I was doing it against! Grace mixed with faith and love poured over me and into me. And all because of Jesus.

Here's a word you can take to heart and depend on: Jesus Christ came into the world to save sinners. I'm proof—*Public Sinner Number One*—of someone who could never have made it apart from sheer mercy. And now he shows me off—evidence of his endless patience—to those who are right on the edge of trusting him forever.[6]

Paul claims no one can surpass his sinful rebellion against God. No one has more right to expect God's distancing, judgment, and condemnation than the man who hunted and killed followers of Jesus. And yet, by the "endless patience" of God, Paul received a radical welcome home. He boldly faced his shadow, all those broken-off, exiled, dismissed, and disgusting parts of himself, and brought them back into himself as he was empowered by the persistent love of God.

Sifting through archaeological rubble, researchers discover shards and scraps left behind by civilizations long since passed. Meticulously, they recreate homes and shelters, tools and toys, and economies and systems. What is most impressive to me, however, is their restoration of ancient artwork, including statues and mosaics broken and shattered by invasions, earthquakes, and the slow erosion of time. Carefully extracted from the often unyielding ground, they collect pieces and fragments of the masterpiece, painstakingly rebuilding and reforging it to its original design. Though shattered by a world bent on destruction, the archeologists' work returns it to all the splendor once intended by the original artist.

In the same way, the Sage finds buried in his boyhood the broken pieces, shards, and lost parts of himself and, together with the Great Restorer, reforges his masterpiece with purpose and hope.

The boy who was ridiculed for being smaller than the other kids gets to come out from hiding. The middle schooler who had his underwear and pants stolen in the locker room is clothed once again. The boy who learned to calm his mother's hysteria and contain his father's wrath is relieved of duty, being allowed to tend to his own heart rather than take care of theirs. The teenager who finds his only solace in porn and masturbation has his desire blessed and loved rather than hated and disparaged. The boy who learned to cut, drink, or have sex in order to numb his pain is asked about his pain and offered comfort rather than merely having his behavior controlled. The rageful young man who found power in his anger gets to drop his fists at the sight of a strong man's kind eyes and melt into a safety long sought but not yet found. The ignored and neglected boy who grew up in an emotional desert finds more than a few drops of water at the well of welcome, attunement, and connection. The younger boy who stepped back from the chaos of his family to wear the leopard costume instead of Superman now gets to don his cape.

All the lost, exiled, broken, confused, buried, hated, scarred, missed, neglected, abused, unfathered, shattered, angry, hopeless, ravaged, weak, powerless, abandoned, and betrayed parts of us can now be returned, restored, and reintegrated.

The Sage is not naive, knowing all too well the parts of himself that have failed. He knows the dark corners of his heart, those places where shame and sin have hidden and festered. He knows his anger and his lust, and he has agreed with Jesus how murderous and adulterous[7] his heart actually is. He has wrestled with the liar that lives within, not excusing his deceit but kindly wondering what fear sits behind the lies, and he cares tenderly for the part of himself afraid of exposure and loss. He feels the pain of childhood neglect and knows the moment he vowed to take care of himself at all costs, shutting everyone else out and locking the door on his heart.

Therefore, the Sage is able to stay with others in the midst of their despair, fear, shame, and hatred because he has explored his own, having done the work of fathering his own heart in the pursuit of the Father. The second-half man has turned towards those parts of himself that, throughout the first half, have remained sequestered into the background. When a man has done the hard work of welcoming home his own broken parts, reintegrating them into himself through the collaborative grace of God, he can then offer that same generosity to others.

COMING HOME

The conversation I had with my boy this morning may sound to some like delusion or psychological gymnastics. Grown men do not often talk about their inner forays into their past, nor readily admit their boyhood fear, shame, or weakness. We are taught to bury the past, move on, and "set our eyes on the goal." But the more time you spend exploring your story in the first half, the more you come to recognize those younger parts of yourself that have been left behind. As a man reclaims those parts of his own inner landscape, he has increasing capacity to tend to those boyhood parts and actively reintegrate them into himself.

The storywork a man does in his first half involves: (1) becoming **aware** that he *has* a story and that the story is one of both divine masterpiece *and* evil's intentional pursuit to steal, kill, and destroy the *imago Dei* in him; (2) slowing down long enough to be **curious** about the story rather than judge, diminish, or dismiss it, and allowing a brotherhood of men access to the story to also be aware and curious; in order for (3) **kindness** to enter the narrative in places where it formerly has not been known, bringing blessing as a weapon of hope to restore that which has been lost. As a result, that first-half man can then take ownership of the story that is yet to be written. This is powerful yet uncommon work among men. Therefore, we have carefully crafted Brotherhood[8] resources and experiences to assist you in this journey.

The task of the second passage is to find the boy within the man and bring him home. This involves:

- Taking the shards of his narrative, blessed and restored as they are from his first half's work, and reintegrating them as part of his true identity, his True Self, thus agreeing with God's delight in the original masterpiece that he is.
- Recollecting his externalized projections and taking responsibility to partner with God to tend to his own needs.
- Identifying the hidden, denied, and exiled parts of himself, those parts that remain untended and in shadow, and inviting them back.
- Entering their dark caves, bringing the light of Life to shine upon them as included parts of his broken self in need of redemption and healing.
- Settling into an existence that extends beyond the limitations of this world, joining the flow of eternity's timeline, "sitting down" in the I AM with full recognition that his being depends solely on the being and existence of God.[9]
- Knowing *his story* is but a part of the Great Story and resting in knowing the Great Hero.

In so doing, he comes home to himself in all the stages of his life, whether past, present, or future. This is what it means to pass the threshold of the second half–to participate in the homecoming to God.

Consider David Benner's wise words:

Christian spirituality involves acknowledging all our part-selves, exposing them to God's love and letting him weave them into the new person he is making. To do this, we must be willing to welcome these ignored parts as full members of the family of self, giving them space at the family table and slowly allowing them to be softened and healed by love and integrated into the whole person we are becoming.[10]

When we invite and welcome those ignored shards of ourselves back, we bring our younger boys to the cross of Christ, asking for his love to overwhelm, envelope, and restore them back to ourselves. The desire of God is to restore the masterpiece so that we more fully reflect the image of Christ as we become more like the men he originally created us to be. As we become Sages, he returns us more and more to our first story.

The scrappy boy who learned how to survive in a non-Edenic world by finding ways to provide for his own needs, whether physical, emotional, relational, or psychological, is welcomed home in the Sage's settled contentment, knowing his "enough" comes from a different and better Father. The second-half man does the hard work of honoring his scrappiness and calming his fears, releasing him from the fear of lack and welcoming him home to internal abundance.

The scared younger part, convinced he must be bigger, better, more important, stronger, more successful, and smarter than others in order to be accepted and loved, is invited by the Sage's inner hospitality to put down his narcissism and take a seat. He is loved for who he is and is freed to find space for himself and others to merely exist.

The Sage speaks to the younger boy in him who has required either/or and black/white thinking in order to find spiritual security and safety in his faith journey, creating space for him to come home to a generous spirituality of a God who cannot be contained. The man who has journeyed through the second passage welcomes him to the great mystery and invites him to the *un*knowing of God.

The boy who has known deep suffering, trauma, and loss finds within the Sage a place to grieve the true nature of his wounds.

There in the place of suffering, he is tended to and cared for by one who does not need him to "get over it"; instead, he is offered the space to collapse with sorrow into the strong and tender arms of another.

The lonely boy in desperate need of a friend finds within the Sage a place to belong when he discovers in solitude the companionship of his own soul. He has re-collected his desperate projections onto others, bringing them back to his own self. He has also put down his personas, freeing him to be the masterpiece of God's original design. In so doing, he makes friends with his younger part and welcomes him home.

The scrappy boy. The scared boy. The either/or boy. The wounded boy. The lonely boy. As long as these exiled and lost boys exist within us, it is our second-half task to find them, bless them, and bring them home to sit at the table of our True Self. There, in the safety of our internal home, touched by the healing hand of Jesus the Great Restorer, the emerging man is reintegrated and welcomed over the threshold and into the Sage.

TWO BRAVE MEN

"But you don't know what I've done! You don't know the darkness that lurks inside me," 47-year-old Robert said as he wrestled with his heart. "I can't accept that story."

"Can you see that boy who lived the story? Do you have a picture of what he looks like in your mind?" I asked.

"Yes," he answered, eyes closed, irritated but quiet. "I know what he looks like."

To get our bearings, I asked, "How old is he, do you think?"

"Seven. I know he's seven," Robert said decisively.

"What does he look like? Where is he?" I wondered.

"He's hiding in the far corner under the bed. He's dirty, disgusting, smelly. He has ripped shorts, no shoes, and no shirt," Robert replied. "He has shorts but no underwear. He never wears underwear because he doesn't like them."

"Why is he hiding?" I asked gently.

"He knows what he did was bad and wrong and *disgusting*," he said, barely able to get the words out, the tissue in his hands disintegrating as he folded and ripped it repeatedly, wringing it in his hands.

"So, he already knows what he did was not good. He doesn't need to be told again. What does he need now?" I asked.

Robert replied, "He's afraid to come out because he's scared he'll get in trouble."

"Does he need to get in trouble for what he did?" I asked.

"No. He's already been in enough trouble. And the dirt and the disgustingness feels bad enough," he insightfully responded.

"So, what does he need now?" I repeated.

Hesitantly, Robert said, "He needs to come out from under the bed."

With tenderness in my voice, I asked, "And where does he want to go?"

"To me. He wants me to hold him." he replied.

"Do you want to hold him?" I asked.

"Yes, I do. But no, he is disgusting, and he smells. He's got all sorts of shit and blood on his face and hands and all over his body," Robert observed. "He's done things, and things have been done to him. He's so nasty."

"Does he need someone to help him clean up and change clothes?" I wondered.

"Probably. He's been like that for a long time, and no one has wanted to come close. Not even me," Robert said through flowing tears.

After Robert caught his breath, I asked, "Would you like to help him now?"

"Yeah. He's been hiding in that corner, reeking of shit and blood and bile for far too long. No one else is going to come for him. I am the only one who can help him," he said, as he took a big heaving breath and put his face in his hands.

Over the next several minutes and through waves of uncontrollable sobs and calm clarity, Robert did the hard work of welcoming his scared, lonely, dirty boy back to himself. For the first time, the man saw the boy with compassionate rather than disgusted eyes, and a visible shift occurred on his face. Jesus sat there on the couch with them, the man and his younger self, and tenderly wiped the scum off his face with a cloth wet by his own tears. I sat in awe and wonder, having just witnessed a holy and tender moment of healing, recovery, and ReStorying.[11]

In the following weeks, Robert unpacked more of this boy's story. And while the details of his life remain his alone to navigate, I am in awe of his pursuit to recover this lost boy and bring him home. The shift in Robert's posture toward himself from disgust and contempt to kindness opened the door for God's healing and love to overwhelm him back to wholeness. For Robert, the exiled boy received the welcome he had been waiting for, and the fractured man took a bold step toward the fullness God originally intended. The masterpiece was slowly being restored.

Another man named Curtis remained quiet for what felt like hours, slowly and silently debating whether he could talk about it or not. At 52 years old, he sat on the precipice of his second half, but he knew he could not enter without addressing a long-exiled part of his heart.

We sat together late into the night in a secluded corner of a retreat center while he unconsciously bit his lip and rocked with the fear of exposure and rejection. Finally, either from courage or desperation, he said, "I've been masturbating since I was 11. For almost 40 years, it's been at least once a day, if not more. And I can't stop. I've tried. Oh God, I've tried! But it never works."

"Thank you for telling me, Curtis. That is very brave," I replied, and then I calmly said, "And I'm still here."

"I've never told anyone," he said, barely looking up.

Curtis had lived almost his entire life with this burning secret. He had never told his wife or even his closest friends, burying his shame in the deepest recesses of his heart. No matter how hard he tried to prevent it, like a werewolf under a full moon, the compulsion rose within him, and he could not keep from being consumed by its power.

"I know now, and I'm honored to be the first. Can you tell me, how did it start?" I asked.

"I discovered it when I was eleven. It just happened one night in bed, rubbing on the sheets, and it felt so good. The rest of my life at the time sucked, totally sucked. Mom had her wine, Dad had his cigarettes, my brother was a complete bully, my sister was sleeping around, and no one seemed to notice I was even there. I was just an inconvenience for everyone. So when I found it, for the first time in a long time, something actually felt good," he admitted.

I could tell Curtis was a good man at heart. I could not imagine how hard it must have been to hold this secret for so long. Clearly, he felt there was a lot at stake.

"No wonder you went back to it," I replied.

"Yeah, of course I did," he said. "On top of that, I got nothing from my dad. Nothing. I was so desperate to feel like a man, and he gave me absolutely nothing. I tried for a while to get his attention, but then I gave up because all I got was his anger and dismissal. My brother got it from him, but not me. And so, I was convinced I was less than a man."

He spoke with clarity and awareness, having already done some good work in his story. But he had never gone this far.

Curtis went on to explain how he had not been athletic as a boy and how small his body felt. Other boys were getting muscles and facial hair, yet he looked like a fifth grader until his sophomore year of high school. Puberty hit him in stages, starting below the belt but then taking years to complete its work elsewhere. As a result, even his brother walloped on him, a readily accessible punching bag by which to take out his anger.

I said, "And erections and ejaculations make an 11-year-old boy feel like a man, don't they?"

"Oh yeah. For that little boy, it was the closest he'd ever come to feeling like a man. So powerful, so raw, so primal," he said, with an edge to his voice.

And then his face turned downwards again, and he covered his eyes with his hand.

"Where did you just go?" I asked.

"I just remembered myself sitting in the bathroom one night. I must have been 12 or something" he whispered. "I felt so alone, so weak, so unseen. I think that day I had masturbated like seven or eight times already just to escape how bad I felt. I wanted to do it one more time before bed, but I couldn't because I'd rubbed my penis raw. It was red and raw like a rug burn, and it was even starting to bleed a little. The skin was literally rubbing off."

He took a few deep breaths and continued, "Even my comfort turned to pain. For the next few days, I had to wrap it in toilet paper to protect it from my jeans. It hurt so much. Bandaids didn't work. They don't stay on parts of your body that always change size, and they hurt to take off. I had no one to tell, no one to help."

"What kind of help do you need?" I asked.

Back to talking about the boy, he replied, "He needs someone to see how much it hurts. His penis, yes, but also his heart," he wisely answered.

"I wonder if every time adult Curtis goes to masturbate now, he needs the same thing," I said.

He looked at me dumbfounded. "What do you mean?" he asked.

"That boy knew he needed to feel like a man. He needed something or someone to fill the emotional void. One night in a normal pubescent moment, his penis answered the question for him, at least in part, and gave him a way to feel like a true man through sexual release. The physical experience became an emotional one. So that desperate boy went hard after it, so hard he rubbed himself raw," I explained. "Now, years later, in moments when the adult Curtis feels emotionally empty, vacant, lonely, or less-than-a-man, he knows where to go to find it...his penis. And every day he needs that reassurance. But what if you gave him something your father could not? What if you gave him the answer he's looking for?"

I leaned forward to make sure he caught my eyes.

"I left him back there, didn't I?" he asked.

"Yes, you did. Of course you did, and you had no way of knowing it. Your scrappy boy found a way to meet his needs. It worked for him then, but it's not working any longer. He's been waiting for you to find him again to tell him he's a man," I replied.

Wide-eyed, he looked at me, and with new awareness, he said, "Once he gets that answer from me he won't have to beat his penis desperate for validation anymore, will he?"

He looked shocked and relieved.

"You are right. His penis can't answer his question. Only you can," I said, as I pointed to his heart.

As we sat there at 2 a.m., Curtis returned to the lost boy inside him, answered his question, and welcomed him back, and he is more ready to enter his second half because he began to recover this lost boy. Now, every time he feels the question rise in his heart, he is able to meet it with a more helpful answer from one who can actually offer it.

THE BOYS AT YOUR MAN'S TABLE

In Matthew 6, Jesus teaches his disciples how to pray, reciting for them what we have come to know as the Lord's Prayer. He begins by saying, "This, then, is how you should pray: 'Our Father in heaven, hallowed be your name, your kingdom come, your will be done, on earth as it is in heaven.'"[12] Jesus instructs us to beseech the Father to make true here and now on earth what is true in his eternal kingdom. For each one of us, there still exists in the mind of God a divine poem written long before the world came into being. Though evil's marauders and vandals have sought to deface, hijack, and lay claim, nothing can separate God's image from his image bearer. As we pray then as Jesus taught, to restore his divine will for this masterpiece on earth, we join the Great Restoration when we gather our exiled parts and welcome them back to sit together with us at the table of our hearts. Indeed, it is the welcome of God back to the original masterpiece he first breathed to life.

The Sage of the second half has come to know the secret of settled contentment, welcoming home that part of himself who no longer seeks to satisfy his hunger or quench his thirst at any other table but his own.

The second-half man has a large space of inner hospitality, welcoming home the lost boy and celebrating his victories, mourning his losses, and finding for him a throne in the room of his own heart.

The Sage's generous spirituality now entertains mystery and expansiveness, holding fast to the unfathomable love of Jesus as he welcomes home the divinely inspired boy.

He weeps, mourns, and explores even the darkest caves of suffering, as he welcomes home the parts of his heart that have suffered significantly yet silently, and he anoints him with the hard-won balm of hope.

The second-half Sage revels in God's company in solitude, looking to his shining face for kindness, care, and peace, as he welcomes home his younger self and befriends him once again.

These internal boys return home, re-collected from their exiled, dismissed, and forgotten places. Time begins to work backwards as these shattered parts once again become more whole. The first-half man gathers other men—other kings—around his table. The Sage's table, however, is now surrounded by *his own men* and *his own boys*, and, for the first time together, they remember what it means to be at home in the Great Masterpiece of God.

The task of the first passage, as the boy becomes a man, is to find the man within the boy and call him forth.

The task of the second passage, as the man becomes a Sage, is to find the boy within the man and bring him home. In so doing, and as we intentionally engage the second half of our journey as men on this earth, we actively participate in the greatest narrative in all history–the restoration of all things. God's promise to a broken world is not to make all new things. His promise is to make *all things new...again.*

QUESTIONS TO CONSIDER AND DISCUSS:

- *Consider each of the names offered for the younger parts living within us: the scrappy boy, the scared boy, the either/or boy, the suffering boy, and the lonely boy. In your life and story, what are you aware of for each? In what ways do you identify with them? How do you not?*
- *From a posture of curiosity rather than judgment, what happened to that boy? What did he have to do to survive?*
- *How might you offer that boy the kindness of God? What does he need from you, the adult part of you, to be welcomed back home?*
- *As you consider your own internal boys gathered at your own internal table, what begins to be possible? What does that homecoming create within you?*
- *What help might you need to find to navigate through this process?*

CONCLUSION
LIVING YOUR UNLIVED LIFE IN THE SECOND HALF

Almost six years ago, I got my first tattoo in Glasgow, Scotland, at the end of the trip with Greg, Bart, and Shae. We all got tattoos, each one different, each one intentional and meaningful for the man who would wear it the rest of his life. For me, it marked the beginning of a new journey, a significant step towards my second half, one where I am purposefully and more consciously living into my meaning and my calling. In the very tender spot on the inside of my right wrist now sits a Celtic knot symbolizing the "Unrelenting Warrior," the twisting lines simultaneously forming an arrow and the sign for infinity.

I put it on my right wrist, my dominant hand, as a symbol of my commitment to fight unceasingly on behalf of the kingdom of God. Everywhere I go, every time I reach to shake a hand, offer help, give directions, click a mouse, stir a pot, stoke a fire, it is *this* hand I extend and *this* intent I bring. At times when I sit in conversations with others, my hands in my lap or on the table, I see the tattoo facing me, and I gently but secretly stroke it to remember my purpose and commitment to God as I engage his people.

Headed into that day at the tattoo studio, I knew what I wanted, and I had known for all the months we prepared for the trip. But at the last minute, something stirred in me, and I knew I needed to add two words to the design. Though I did not yet fully understand it, I knew it would not be complete without the words "Bard King" written underneath. Thankfully, the artist agreed.

Since the tattoo, I have sat many times with Jesus asking about those words. They come from the Stephen Lawhead books[1] I previously mentioned, referencing the mighty man once named Myrddin Emrys, the counselor to famous King Arthur of legend. While all of us know what a king is, a bard of ancient England is the wise man who reads the text of life, listens to the Spirit of God, and intimately knows the remedies offered in the herbs of the earth. He speaks the language of friend and foe alike and communes with Jesus through prayer and petition. He holds the stories and histories of the people, singing them in the king's court and over the pre-battle war host to offer the courage that comes from remembering past victories and the omnipotent hand of God. Once a king himself, Myrddin Emrys more deeply understood his purpose to uphold the high kingship of Arthur, and soon he became known as the Sage of the land. Since first reading about him as a teen, he has been my model, my example, my mentor, and my aim in my masculine journey: the Bard King. You likely know of him as Merlin.

For the past six years, this tattoo has been a daily reminder of my purpose. In moments when I have extended my hand in harm, whether intentional or not, I am confronted with a visual invitation to return to the calling I know God designed for me. I need this reminder often. In fact, I need it every day.

In a few days I will leave the Irish coast and return to suburban America. Today the clouds are low, and though it is not raining, everything is wet. Earth and sky are near to one another, and I keep the fire blazing to keep the chill out of the room. This place has been my hermitage, my hut, my home for the past several weeks, and no one but I will know all that these walls and shores witnessed of my own second-half wrestlings. But more than ever before, I have found him, I have found *them*, the orphaned boys inside me who have waited for my invitation to come home. More than laboring to write this book, this month has been a labor of my own heart. I will return a changed man.

I will take two buses and two trains to make my way to Dublin before taking two planes to return to my home in Colorado. But before I leave Ireland, I have one more important task—I am getting another tattoo. The first one on my right arm was inked in the camaraderie of my brotherhood of men. This one, however, comes with the restored fellowship of my returned boys. For while on my right arm is the symbol of my *purpose* and *calling*, I now mark my left arm with the symbol of my *identity*. What I am called to do on the right, and who I am called to be on the left. Two arms extended together to bring the fullness of who I am—as best I can while I walk the earth—to the world.

Buy me a coffee or a beer (better yet, a Guinness!), and I will show you and tell you all about them.

IT'S UP TO YOU

My friend, the choice is yours. Will you walk the path of the Sage? Will you intentionally approach the threshold of the second passage with circumspect, humility, purpose, and will? It is up to you to do the work and become the Sage God designed you to be. You are the only one who can walk it, and you are the only one who can keep you from it. Your own fear, your own apathy, your own resignation, your own addiction, or your own lack of courage, compassion, or imagination stand between you and your True Self.

The fact is, you are going to age regardless of what you do. Your march towards your eventual departure from this earth cannot be halted. But you get to decide what kind of journey it is going to be.

Is it any wonder, in a discussion about who is greatest in the kingdom, Jesus admonishes us to become like children once again? The Gospel of Matthew tells us,

> At that time the disciples came to Jesus and asked, 'Who, then, is the greatest in the kingdom of heaven?' He called a little child to him and, placing the child among them, he said: 'Truly I tell you, unless you change and become like little children, you will never enter the kingdom of heaven. Therefore, whoever *takes the lowly position of this child* is the greatest in the kingdom of heaven. And *whoever welcomes one such child in my name welcomes me*.[2]

We must return to the little boy living in the man and father him home. It is only as you come to the end of your first-half strength, resources, cunning, and power that you can occupy the position of the child. Ultimately, it is the return to the child that embodies the second half of a man's life.

Let us return to where we began, a vision for a world of Sages. Together, as a generation of men, we have both the opportunity and the responsibility to alter the course of history by embracing the high calling of God to fully become the men he designed and intended. We have it within us to bring heaven just a little closer to earth, starting first with the transformation of ourselves, and then our families, our communities, and, ultimately, our world. Let us not just get older, but instead, let us become the Gandalfs, Yodas, Dumbledores, Elis, Nathans, and Jethros of our time.

May this blessing by the wise John O'Donohue be a benediction to your work, and may it cover you on your onward journey.

FOR OLD AGE

May the light of your soul mind you.
May all your worry and anxiousness about your age
Be transfigured

May you be given wisdom for the eyes of your soul
To see this as a time of gracious harvesting.
May you have the passion to heal what has hurt you,
And allow it to come closer and become one with you.

May you have great dignity,
Sense how free you are;
Above all, may you be given the wonderful gift
Of meeting the eternal light that is within you.

May you be blessed;
And may you find a wonderful love
In your self for your self.[3]

ACKNOWLEDGMENTS

I firmly believe a man becomes a man through other men, and the man I have become is because of the few Sages who have seen beyond my masks and into my heart. Your bold love has invited me over and over to come back to myself, and I am forever grateful. To Ben McComb, Mark Rehfuss, Dan Allender, Steve Call, O'Donnell Day, Roy Barsness, Craig Glass, Stephen Lawhead, and Merlin, I am who I am because of you.

Additionally, it has been through the deep community of men of Restoration Project I have found the courage to look at my own story and pursue my own boys. From the beginning, we have endeavored to heal our wounds, know our God, and restore the world. It has been a journey marked by high peak victories and dark valley failures. To all the men, far too numerous to list by name here, who have been part of my journey, I thank you and honor you. My greatest wealth is found in my relationships with you. Thank you.

To Greg Daley, Bart Lillie, and Shae McCowen, the three brave men who adventured with me into the Scottish Highlands six years ago, I thank you. Greg, thanks for planning the trip and for being a comrade in the battle for men's hearts, including my own. Shae and Bart, thanks for saying "yes!" to everything we had crafted for that experience and all the other adventures before and after that trip. While the physical journey in Scotland was epic, the spiritual journey proved far more important. What we started together there has continued to broaden and deepen in my soul. To all three of you, thank you for continuing to pursue my heart. WTFB.

My deepest and sincerest gratitude to the Restoration Project Board who blessed and financially supported my journey to Ireland to write this book. Your gift of space, time, and focus allowed me to do the hard internal work necessary to even *begin* to consider putting these feeble thoughts down on paper. Thank you.

Similarly, to the staff of Restoration Project, who honored my departure and held the entire organization together in my stead, I thank you. Jesse French, Christina Vink, Cody Buriff, Kevin Armstrong, and Jeremy Williamson...you are the greatest team on the planet, and it is a tremendous privilege to be counted as one among you. OSFD. Thank you.

To the staff at Restoration Counseling, who blessed this project and sent me away while you continued to hold the stories of so many in your care while simultaneously pressing forward in our work and organization, I know my absence cost you, and I am grateful. A special thanks to Beth Bruno, Tracy Johnson, Lindy Pearson, and Christina Vink for offering kind and bold leadership. To Katelyn O'Grady, Lisa Russell, Kevala Kenna, Cris Flippen, CJ Rithner, Lynsey Crevier, Alex Murphy, Leslie Coy, Nicole Clifton, Reid Fuller, Becky Young, Jeremy Williamson, Julie Kittredge, Michael Krommendyk, and Valerie Rausseo, a big and heartfelt thank you.

My deepest gratitude to the Michael Cameron Dempsey Fund for your generous grant in support of this work. May Michael's legacy be honored and remembered through the impact of these words in the lives of men around the world. Thank you.

To Brian and Philomena, my wonderful Irish hosts, to the residents of Dun Chaoin, Ireland, and the patrons and staff of Kruger's Bar, a heartfelt thank you for your hospitality, warm fires, and many drafts of Guinness.

To Susan Tucker, my generous, kind, meticulous, and thoughtful editor, I owe a tremendous debt of gratitude. The way you have engaged me and this manuscript has been both bold and tender. Your way with words, concepts, and punctuation astounds me.

Thank you for pouring over this work. It would not be what it is without you. Thank you!

And to Beth, my dearest love, my life-companion, my heart. Words are insufficient to express my gratitude and awe for all you have offered throughout my life. You have always blessed my boys and my man, even when I have not or could not. Your kindness has been the very balm of my healing and continues to offer me hope that one day I can truly be the man God designed for you. Thank you for sending me to Ireland. Thank you for being the first to read the book. Thank you for your gentle suggestions and curious invitations that have made this work more than I could have alone. You are, and always will be, my most trusted and loved one on earth. Thank you.

BIBLIOGRAPHY

- AARP. "History." May 10, 2010. https://www.aarp.org/about-aarp/company/info-2016/history.html.
- Arrien, Angeles. *The Second Half of Life: Opening the Eight Gates of Wisdom.* Boulder, CO: Sounds True, 2007.
- Benner, David G. *The Gift of Being Yourself: The Sacred Call to Self-Discovery.* Downers Grove, IL: InterVarsity Press, 2015.
- Bruno, Chris. *Man Maker Project.* Eugene, OR: Resource Publications, 2015.
- Campbell, Joseph. *The Hero's Journey.* New York: Joseph Campbell Foundation, 2020. https://www.jcf.org/works/titles/the-heros-journey-book/.
- Campbell, Joseph. *The Hero with a Thousand Faces.* New York: Joseph Campbell Foundation, 2020. https://www.jcf.org/works/titles/the-hero-with-a-thousand-faces/.

- Center for Disease Control and Prevention. "Loneliness and Social Isolation Linked to Serious Health Conditions." April 29, 2021. https://www.cdc.gov/aging/publications/features/lonely-older-adults.html.
- Chesterton, G.K. *Orthodoxy.* San Francisco, CA: Ignatius Press, 2021.
- Data Commons. "United States." Accessed May 1, 2022. https://datacommons.org/place/country/USA.
- Dubov, Nissan Dovid. "Tzimtzum." Accessed January 19, 2022. https://www.chabad.org/library/article_cdo/aid/361884.
- Early Church History. "Longevity in the Ancient World." Accessed January 9, 2022. https://earlychurchhistory.org/daily-life/longevity-in-the-ancient-world/.
- Eldredge, John. *Fathered by God: Learning What Your Dad Could Never Teach You.* Nashville, TN: Thomas Nelson, 2009.
- Frankl, Viktor. *Man's Search for Meaning.* Boston, MA: Beacon Press, 2006.
- Glass, Craig. *Noble Journey: The Quest for a Lasting Legacy.* Monument, CO: Peregrine Ministries, 2017.
- Grudem, Wayne. *Systematic Theology: An Introduction to Biblical Doctrine.* Grand Rapids, MI: Zondervan, 1994.
- Hicks, Robert. *Masculine Journey: Understanding the Six Stages of Manhood.* Colorado Springs, CO: NavPress, 1993.
- Hillman, James. *Insearch: Psychology and Religion.* Thompson, CT: Spring Publications, 2015.
- Hollis, James. *Living an Examined Life: Wisdom for the Second Half of the Journey.* Boulder, CO: Sounds True, 2018.
- —. *The Middle Passage: From Misery to Meaning in Midlife.* Toronto: Inner City Books, 1993.
- Killam, Kasley. "To Combat Loneliness, Promote Social Health." *Scientific American,* January 23, 2018.

https://www.scientificamerican.com/article/to-combat-loneliness-promote-social-health1.
- Lawhead, Stephen. *Pendragon Cycle*. Wheaton, IL: Crossway. Books, 1987.
- L'Engle, Madeleine. *A Circle of Quiet*. New York: Crosswicks, Ltd., 1972.
- Lesté-Lasserre, Christa. "Young Male Elephants Rein in Aggression If Older Males Are Nearby." *New Scientist*, December 22, 2021. https://www.newscientist.com/article/2302675.
- Lewis, C.S. *A Grief Observed*. New York: Harper Collins, 1961.
- —. *Mere Christianity*. New York: Harper Collins, 1952.
- —. *The Last Battle*. New York: HarperTrophy, 2000.
- —. *The Lion, the Witch, and the Wardrobe*. New York: Macmillan, 1950.
- —. *Weight of Glory*. New York: Harper Collins, 1949.
- Marshall, Bruce. *The World, the Flesh, and Father Smith*. Garden City, NY: Image Books, 1957.
- Merton, Thomas. *New Seeds of Contemplation*. New York: New Directions, 1961.
- Milliken, Caleb. "Rites of Passage for Michael Milliken." Accessed January 13, 2022. https://www.indiegogo.com/projects/rites-of-passage-for-michael-milliken.
- Moore, Robert, and Douglas Gillette. *King, Warrior, Magician, Lover: Rediscovering the Archetypes of the Mature Masculine*. San Francisco, CA: Harper Collins, 1990.
- Morley, Patrick. *Seven Seasons of the Man in the Mirror*. Grand Rapids, MI: Zondervan, 2010.
- Nouwen, Henri J.M. *The Wounded Healer*. New York: Doubleday, 1972.
- —. *Turn My Mourning into Dancing: Finding Hope in Hard Times*. Nashville, TN: Thomas Nelson, 2001.

- O'Donohue, John. *To Bless the Space Between Us: A Book of Blessings.* New York: Doubleday, 2008.
- Palmer, Parker. *Let Your Life Speak: Listening for the Voice of Vocation.* San Francisco, CA: Jossey-Bass, 2000.
- Park, Laura Hackett. "Shalom." Kansas City, MO: Arrowhead Music Publishing, 2021.
- Pasricha, Neil. "Why Retirement Is a Flawed Concept." *Harvard Business Review,* April 13, 2016. https://hbr.org/2016/04/why-retirement-is-a-flawed-concept.
- Pentecost, George. *The Angel in the Marble, and Other Papers.* London: Hodder and Stoughton, 1883.
- Peterson, Eugene. *The Message.* Colorado Springs, CO: NavPress, 2018.
- Plotkin, Bill. *Soulcraft: Crossing Into the Mysteries of Nature and the Psyche.* Novato, CA: New World Library, 2003.
- Pomeroy, Claire. "Loneliness Is Harmful to Our Nation's Health." *Scientific American,* March 20, 2019. https://blogs.scientificamerican.com/observations/loneliness-is-harmful-to-our-nations-health/.
- Precept Austin. "Believers Are God's Masterpiece, His Poiema." January 31, 2021. https://www.preceptaustin.org/gods_masterpiece-poiema_greek_word_study.
- Ro, Christine. "Why the Sandwich Generation Is So Stressed Out." January 29, 2021. https://www.bbc.com/worklife/article/20210128-why-the-sandwich-generation-is-so-stressed-out.
- Rohr, Richard. *Falling Upward: A Spirituality for the Two Halves of Life.* San Francisco, CO: Jossey-Bass, 2011.
- ———. *The Naked Now: Learning to See as the Mystics See.* New York: The Crossroad Publishing Company, 2009.
- Roosevelt, Theodore. "Citizenship in a Republic." Transcript of speech delivered at the Sorbonne, Paris,

France, April 23, 1910. https://www.americanrhetoric.com/speeches/teddyrooseveltcitizenshipinrepublicarena.htm.
- Schnachter-Shalomi, Zalman, and Ronald S. Miller. 2014. *From Age-ing to Sage-ing: A Revolutionary Approach to Growing Older.* New York: Grand Central Publishing.
- Sheehy, Gail. *Understanding Men's Passages: Discovering the New Map of Men's Lives.* New York: Ballantine Books, 1999.
- Smith, Douglas A., and Kenneth F. Murphy. *Thriving in the Second Half of Life.* Columbus, OH: White Pine Mountain, 2020.
- Snyder, Morgan. *Becoming a King: The Path to Restoring the Heart of a Man.* Nashville, TN: Thomas Nelson, 2020.
- Social Security Administration. "Historical Background and Development of Social Security." Accessed January 15, 2022. https://www.ssa.gov/history/briefhistory3.html.
- Statista. "Estimated expenses of the U.S. motion picture and video industries from 2007 to 2019." Accessed January 18, 2022. https://www.statista.com/statistics/185312.
- Stein, Murray. *In Midlife: A Jungian Perspective.* Asheville, NC: Chiron Publications, 2014.
- Tolkein, J.R.R. *The Fellowship of the Ring.* New York: Harper Collins, 2004.
- Van Biema, David. "Should Christians Convert Muslims?" *Time,* June 30, 2003.
- West, Christopher. *Fill These Hearts: God, Sex, and the Universal Longing.* New York: Image, 2012.
- Willard, Dallas. *The Divine Conspiracy: Rediscovering Our Hidden Life in God.* New York: Harper Collins, 1997.
- Willis, Timothy. "Elders in the Old Testament Community." *Leaven* 2, no. 1 (1992). https://digitalcommons.pepperdine.edu/cgi/viewcontent.cgi?article=2008&context=leaven.

- Wilson, C., and B. Moulton. "Loneliness Among Older Adults: A National Survey of Adults 45+." *AARP The Magazine,* September 2010. https://assets.aarp.org/rgcenter/general/loneliness_2010.pdf.

NOTES

INTRODUCTION

1. John O'Donohue, *To Bless the Space Between Us: A Book of Blessings* (New York: Doubleday, 2008), 48-49.
2. Chris Bruno, *Man Maker Project* (Eugene, OR: Resource Publications, 2015).
3. These three core conditions are the foundation upon which all Restoration Project experiences are built.
4. Restoration Counseling (www.restorationcounselingnoco.com)
5. Restoration Project (www.restorationproject.net)
6. RIchard Rohr, *Falling Upward: A Spirituality for the Two Halves of Life* (San Francisco, CA: Jossey-Bass, 2011), 89.
7. Bruno, *Man Maker Project,* 2015.
8. Most notably, Richard Rohr, *Falling Upward,* and James Hollis, *The Middle Passage: From Misery to Meaning in Midlife.*
9. G.K. Chesterton, *Orthodoxy* (San Francisco, CA: Ignatius Press, 2021), 59.

1. MEETING GANDALF, THE HERO'S HERO

1. According to recent data, the life expectancy for an American male in 2021 is 78.79 years. "United States," Data Commons, Accessed May 1, 2022, https://datacommons.org/place/country/USA.
2. Viktor Frankl, *Man's Search for Meaning* (Boston, MA: Beacon Press, 2006), loc. 26 of 2041, Kindle.
3. James Hollis, *The Middle Passage: From Misery to Meaning in Midlife* (Toronto: Inner City Books, 1993), 94.
4. Hollis, *Middle Passage*, 7.
5. In this description, I have shortened and adapted the hero's journey significantly. For more, see Joseph Campbell, *The Hero's Journey* (New York: Joseph Campbell Foundation, 2020).
6. I should note epic stories are also full of female heroes who face similar battles against darkness. Likewise, on their quests, they also require a guide to set them on the right path.
7. A "Man Year" is the term I use in the *Man Maker Project*. It describes the year of transition from boy to man and the father's role to intentionally call forth the man from within the boy and invite him to the company of men.

2. THE MASCULINE DESTINATION

1. "History," AARP, May 10, 2010, https://www.aarp.org/about-aarp/company/info-2016/history.html.
2. Neil Pasricha, "Why Retirement Is a Flawed Concept," *Harvard Business Review*, April 13, 2016, https://hbr.org/2016/04/why-retirement-is-a-flawed-concept.
3. "Historical Background and Development of Social Security," Social Security Administration, accessed January 15, 2022, https://www.ssa.gov/history/briefhistory3.html.
4. By this, I specifically mean financial privileges, which are the result of other privileges I have merely by being a white male. To further explore this would require an entire other book.
5. For quick reference on generations: Greatest (born 1910-1924); Silent (born 1925-1945); Boomer (1946-1964); Generation X (born 1965-1979); Millennial/Generation Y (born 1980-1995); Generation Z (born 1995-2010); Generation Alpha (born after 2010).
6. Christa Lesté-Lasserre, "Young Male Elephants Rein in Aggression If Older Males Are Nearby," *New Scientist,* December 22, 2021, https://www.newscientist.com/article/2302675.
7. Rohr, *Falling Upward*, 111.
8. New American Standard Bible; italics added.
9. Rohr, *Falling Upward,* 123-124.
10. New International Version.
11. "Longevity in the Ancient World," Early Church History, accessed January 9, 2022, https://earlychurchhistory.org/daily-life/longevity-in-the-ancient-world.
12. Luke 2, after Jesus is left behind at the temple, is the last mention of Joseph. Some traditions tell us Joseph was already an older man (by ancient Near East standards) when he married Mary. Deductive reasoning tells us he died shortly thereafter, which, given a man's expected lifespan, makes perfect sense.
13. There are dozens of mentions of elders in the Old Testament, far too many to enumerate here. See Timothy Willis, "Elders in the Old Testament Community," *Leaven*, Vol. 2, Iss. 1, Article 4 (1992). https://digitalcommons.pepperdine.edu/leaven/vol2/iss1/4
14. Adapted from Willis, "Elders," 11.
15. Joseph Campbell, *The Hero with a Thousand Faces* (New York: Joseph Campbell Foundation, 2020), 28.
16. Henri J.M. Nouwen, *The Wounded Healer* (New York: Doubleday, 1972), 67.
17. Dallas Willard, *The Divine Conspiracy* (New York: Harper Collins, 1997), 22.

3. THE DIVINE MASTERPIECE

1. NASB; italics added.
2. NIV; italics added.
3. Psalm 139:13-16, NIV.
4. Ephesians 1:5-6, New Living Translation; italics added.
5. NLT; italics added.

6. "Believers Are God's Masterpiece, His Poemia," Precept Austin, January 31, 2021, https://www.preceptaustin.org/gods_masterpiece-poiema_greek_word_study.
7. NIV.
8. John 10:10, NIV.
9. C.S. Lewis, *The Lion, the Witch, and the Wardrobe* (New York: Macmillan, 1950), 75; Italics added.
10. Parker Palmer, *Let Your Life Speak: Listening for the Voice of Vocation* (San Francisco, CA: Jossey-Bass, 2000), loc. 144-145 of 1030, Kindle.
11. Referring to Psalm 147:3 and Isaiah 61.
12. Many men struggle to find both of these. I refer you to Restoration Counseling (https://restory.life) for a team of highly qualified and kind storywork counselors. I also refer you to my book *Brotherhood Primer* and to the Brotherhood Project at Restoration Project (https://www.restorationproject.net/brotherhood).

4. THE FIRST PASSAGE OF A MAN'S LIFE

1. Bruno, *Man Maker Project*, loc. 283 of 4344, Kindle.
2. Caleb Milliken, "*Rites of Passage for Michael Milliken,*" Indiegogo.com, Accessed January 13, 2022, https://www.indiegogo.com/projects/rites-of-passage-for-michael-milliken.
3. A complete exploration into this topic and rite of passage process can be found in my book *Man Maker Project* (Bruno, 2015) and Restoration Project's work with fathers (restorationproject.net).
4. George Pentecost, *The Angel in the Marble, and Other Papers* (London: Holder and Stoughton, 1883), 12.
5. See Chapter 1 of *Man Maker* for a deeper description of this mess.
6. The list here is far too extensive for me to fully enumerate. However, to name a few, it includes narcissism, depression, violence, lack of emotional intelligence, abdication, power-hunger, anger, absence, and verbal/physical/mental/spiritual/emotional/financial/etc. abuse of others.
7. NASB.
8. Bruno, *Man Maker Project*, 2015.
9. Or father figure. Masculinity can be bestowed on boys and men of any age by any man. While the primary responsibility for this falls on the shoulders of the boy's father, when he is either absent or unavailable, other men can step in to surrogately initiate. I have known grandfathers, uncles, brothers, and even older friends who stand in for missing fathers. And, even though the physical transition through adolescence into adulthood may have happened years ago, I have known grown men who seek initiation from their own fathers. It is never too late.

5. THE MAN OF THE FIRST HALF

1. See Joseph Cambell's *The Hero with a Thousand Faces* for a brilliant and exhaustive exposition on the "monomyth," the singular storyline that all myths and epic stories follow.

2. See John 1.
3. "Estimated expenses of the U.S. motion picture and video industries from 2007 to 2019," Statista, Accessed January 18, 2022, https://www.statista.com/statistics/185312.
4. Theodore Roosevelt, "Citizenship in a Republic,", transcript of address delivered at the Sorbonne, Paris, France, April 23, 1910, https://www.americanrhetoric.com/speeches/teddyrooseveltcitizenshipinrepublicarena.htm.
5. Morgan Snyder, *Becoming a King: The Path to Restoring the Heart of a Man* (Nashville, TN: Thomas Nelson, 2021), xvi.
6. C.S. Lewis, *Weight of Glory* (New York: Harper Collins, 1949), 26.
7. Namely John Eldredge in *Fathered by God* (2009), Robert Hicks in *Masculine Journey* (1993), Joseph Campbell in The *Hero with a Thousand Faces* (2020), Robert Moore and Douglas Gillette in *King, Warrior, Magician, Lover* (1990), and Patrick Morley in *Seven Seasons of the Man in the Mirror* (2010).
8. This phrasing is attributed to Henry David Thoreau.
9. Craig Glass is the founder of Peregrine Ministries, a very like-minded ministry everyone should know. To learn more about him, visit peregrineministries.org.
10. Gail Sheehy, *Understanding Men's Passages: Discovering the New Map of Men's Lives* (New York: Ballantine Books, 1999), 97.
11. Thomas Merton, *New Seeds of Contemplation* (New York: New Directions, 1961), 302.
12. Rohr, *Falling Upward*, loc. 478 of 3008, Kindle.

6. FAILED PROJECTIONS

1. Hollis, *Middle Passage*, 28.
2. Nouwen, *Wounded Healer*, 84.
3. Hollis, *Middle Passage*, 34.
4. Pasricha, "Why Retirement Is a Flawed Concept."
5. Pasricha, "Why Retirement Is a Flawed Concept."
6. Rohr, *Falling Upward*, 113.
7. Frankl, *Man's Search for Meaning*, 109; italics original.
8. Angeles Arrien, *The Second Half of Life: Opening the Eight Gates of Wisdom* (Boulder, CO: Sounds True, 2007), 4.

7. PERSONAS: THE MASKS WE WEAR

1. Throughout my childhood, I heard these words repeated over and over. My mother latched onto them with a fervor more psychological than spiritual. Personally, after a lifetime of walking with Jesus, I firmly believe in God's near and present voice, speaking to us gently, tending to our broken hearts, offering wisdom in moments of decision and clarity in moments of confusion. I have witnessed first-hand the miraculous power of God, and I have come to understand the commitment my mother held to the fulfillment of this prophecy over me had far more to do with her own unlived life than God's directions for mine.

2. Douglas A. Smith and Kenneth F. Murphy, *Thriving in the Second Half of Life* (Columbus, OH: White Pine Mountain, 2020), 31.
3. Palmer, *Let Your Life Speak,* loc. 84 of 1030, Kindle.
4. For more information about the intensives I lead, visit https://www.restory.life/intensives.
5. Hollis, *Middle Passage*, 76.
6. Palmer, *Let Your Life Speak,* loc. 145 of 1030, Kindle.
7. Nouwen, *Wounded Healer*, 76.
8. Nouwen, *Wounded Healer*, 84.

8. MIDLIFE

1. Christine Ro, "Why the 'Sandwich Generation' is so Stressed Out," BBC, January 28, 2021, https://www.bbc.com/worklife/article/20210128-why-the-sandwich-generation-is-so-stressed-out.
2. Craig Glass, *Noble Journey* (Monument, CO: Peregrine Ministries, 2017), 195. And yes, it is the same wise Craig I wrote about several chapters ago.
3. Palmer, *Let Your Life Speak*, loc. 52 of 1030, Kindle.
4. Palmer, *Let Your Life Speak,* loc. 79 of 1030, Kindle.
5. Murray Stein, *In Midlife: A Jungian Perspective* (Asheville: Chiron Publications, 2014), 27.

9. COMING TO THE END OF OURSELVES

1. I learned about this in an American Indian unit at school. *Pemmican* is a snack made of ground meat and ground fruit powder. Unsure of the sanitary nature of meat, not to mention how my mother would respond if I asked for raw meat, I made my own version out of oats, nuts, peanut butter, and coconut flakes.
2. Rohr, *Falling Upward*, 67.
3. Rohr, *Falling Upward*, 42.
4. Bill Plotkin, *Soulcraft: Crossing Into the Mysteries of Nature and Psyche* (Novato, CA: New World Library, 2003).
5. Rohr, *Falling Upward*, 46.
6. Genesis 2:24.
7. A more thorough description and process can be found in the *Brotherhood Primer*, ideal for a small group of men to go through this journey together. Telling his story to a group of men is a powerful experience every man should have.
8. Hollis, *Middle Passage*, 8.
9. C.S. Lewis, *Mere Christianity* (New York: Harper Collins, 1952), 136-137.
10. James Hollis, *Living an Examined Life: Wisdom for the Second Half of the Journey* (Boulder, CO: Sounds True, 2018), 10.
11. Rohr, *Falling Upward*, 97.
12. Hollis, *Middle Passage,* 42.
13. Rohr, *Falling Upward*, 48.
14. NIV.

15. O'Donohue, *To Bless the Space Between Us*, 48.
16. O'Donohue, *To Bless the Space Between Us*, 49.

III. THE SAGE OF THE SECOND HALF

1. From Rainer Maria Rilke's poem, "The Dark Hours of my Being" in *Book of Hours: Love Poems to God*, as quoted in Douglas A. Smith and Kenneth F Murphy, *Thriving in the Second Half of Life* (Columbus, OH: White Pine Mountain, 2020), 30.
2. Arrien, *The Second Half of Life*, 4.
3. C.S. Lewis, *The Last Battle* (New York: Macmillan, 1956), 171.

10. THE SAGE'S ENOUGH: SETTLED CONTENTMENT

1. Philippians 4:11-13, NIV; italics added.
2. Luke 12:22-31.
3. Rohr, *Falling Upward*, 124; italics original.
4. For more information, see https://www.restorationproject.net/back-country-girls-backpacking.
5. Zalman Schnachter-Shalomi and Ronal Miller, *From Age-ing to Sage-ing: A Revolutionary Approach to Growing Older* (New York: Grand Central Publishing, 2014), 26.
6. For many Christian men, *desire* is equated with *lust*. The moment a man experiences desire, especially sexual desire, he is told to eliminate it, move away from it, and in fact, kill it. But desire cannot be killed because it is holy and God-breathed. While these earthly desires can be hijacked, they themselves are not the enemy. The wise man listens to his desire and therein finds his heart for God.
7. Bruce Marshall, *The World, he Flesh, and Father Smith* (Garden City, NY: Image Books, 1957), 114. Over the past several decades, this quote has been misattributed to G.K. Chesterton, when in fact it came from this mid-century novel originally published in 1945.
8. Christopher West, *Fill These Hearts: God, Sex, and the Universal Longing* (New York: Image, 2012), 42, italics original.
9. West, *Fill These Hearts*, 42.
10. Psalm 16:5-11, NIV.
11. Psalm 27:13, NIV.
12. Christopher West refers to these two poles as the addict and the stoic. West, *Fill These Hearts*, 42.
13. John 4:32, 34, NIV.

11. THE SAGE'S WELCOME: A SPACIOUS INNER HOSPITALITY

1. James Hillman, *Insearch: Psychology and Religion* (Thompson, CT: Spring Publications, 2015), loc. 287 of 1844, Kindle.
2. And if you have, I am sorry. You can join us in the car to let your laughter and expletives fly free.
3. John 3:30, NIV.
4. NASB.
5. Philippians 3:4-9, NIV.
6. John Eldredge, *Fathered by God: Learning What Your Dad Could Never Teach You* (Nashville: Thomas Nelson, 2009), 197-198.
7. Nissan Dovid Dubov, "Tzimtzum," Chabad.org, Accessed January 19, 2022, https://www.chabad.org/library/article_cdo/aid/361884/jewish/Tzimtzum.htm.
8. Hillman, *Insearch: Psychology and Religion*, 287.
9. Nouwen, *Wounded Healer*, 88.
10. Eldredge, *Fathered by God*, 201.

12. THE SAGE'S GREAT GOD: GENEROUS SPIRITUALITY

1. Wayne Grudem, *Systematic Theology: An Introduction to Biblical Doctrine* (Grand Rapids, MI: Zondervan, 1994).
2. At that time, we were also highly influenced by John Piper's book *Desiring God,* and then later *Don't Waste Your Life.*
3. David Van Biema, "Should Christians Convert Muslims," *Time*, Vol. 161, No. 26, June 30, 2003.
4. C.S. Lewis, *A Grief Observed* (New York: Harper Collins, 1961), 10.
5. Lewis, *A Grief Observed*, 29.
6. Isaiah 55: 8-9, NIV.
7. Arrien, *The Second Half of Life*, 17.
8. New Revised Standard Version.
9. Romans 11: 33-34, NIV.
10. Rohr, *Falling Upward*, 10.
11. Do not let the word 'mystic' scare you off. It simply means *"one who has moved from mere belief systems or belonging systems to actual inner experience."* (Richard Rohr, *The Naked Now: Learning to See as the Mystics See* (New York: The Crossroad Publishing Company, 2009), 30); italics original.
12. My friend and colleague, Tracy Johnson, has much more brilliance to add to the conversation about liminality. Tracy, please write that book. We all need your wisdom.
13. Merton, *New Seeds of Contemplation*, 302-303.
14. Philippians 3:14, NIV.

13. THE SAGE'S DEATH: THE CRUCIBLE OF SUFFERING

1. The term "national staff" refers to those from the local country who had converted to Christianity and then became missionaries to their own people, working with us on our team.
2. J.R.R. Tolkein, *Fellowship of the Ring* (New York: Harper Collins, 2004), 59.
3. Romans 5:3-5, NIV.
4. Hollis, *Middle Passage*, 19.
5. James 1:2-4, NIV.
6. Yes, women can be addicted to pornography too.
7. Reader be warned: there are several "experts" in the field of sexual addiction recovery. In my work as a therapist with hundreds of men in this area, I have found many of these programs to not only be unhelpful, but actually to exacerbate the harm. The focus is on behavior and sin management rather than a deep engagement with the story of the addicted person. I have stories upon stories. If you find yourself or others in this situation, please be thoughtful and careful in your selection of counselors or programs, and feel free to contact Restoration Counseling for assistance in finding help.
8. Henri Nouwen, *Turn My Mourning into Dancing: Finding Hope in Hard Times* (Nashville: Thomas Nelson, 2001), 10-11.
9. Nouwen, *Turn My Mourning into Dancing*, 12.
10. Hollis, *Middle Passage*, 39.

14. THE SAGE'S COMPANION: FROM LONELINESS TO SOLITUDE

1. According to the 2016 Irish census, https://www.cso.ie/en/index.html.
2. "Loneliness and Social Isolation Linked to Serious Health Conditions," Centers for Disease Control and Prevention, last reviewed April 29, 2021, https://www.cdc.gov/aging/publications/features/lonely-older-adults.html.
3. Kasley Killam, "To Combat Loneliness, Promote Social Health," *Scientific American*, January 23, 2018, https://www.scientificamerican.com/article/to-combat-loneliness-promote-social-health1.
4. Claire Pomeroy, "Loneliness is Harmful to Our Nation's Health," *Scientific American*, March 20, 2019, https://blogs.scientificamerican.com/observations/loneliness-is-harmful-to-our-nations-health.
5. C. Wilson and B. Moulton, "Loneliness Among Older Adults: A National Survey of Adults 45+," AARP The Magazine, September 2010, https://assets.aarp.org/rgcenter/general/loneliness_2010.pdf.
6. Accountability is not designed to keep us *from* sin. No one can do that. Any man who has attempted to "be kept accountable" knows it simply does not work. True accountability is not about keeping us from sin and our second story, but rather it reminds us of who we truly are in our first story. A true brother is a champion of

the masterpiece of his friend, holding faith with him in his first story. This is what it means to have a Jonathan-David relationship, as noted in 2 Samuel 1:26.
7. See Restoration Project's multitude of resources and experiences designed to create and deepen true brotherhood. https://www.restorationproject.net/brotherhood.
8. Nouwen, *Turn My Mourning into Dancing*, 75-76.
9. NIV.
10. Exodus 34:29-35.
11. Merton, *New Seeds of Contemplation*, 48; italics original.
12. Psalm 62:5, NRSV.
13. David G. Benner, *The Gift of Being Yourself: The Sacred Call to Self-Discovery* (Downers Grove, IL: InterVarsity Press, 2015), 86.
14. Here are my favorite three: *Invitation to Silence and Solitude* by Ruth Haley Barton, *The Way of the Heart* by Henri Nouwen, and *The Practice of the Presence of God* by Brother Lawrence. Clearly, there are many more than I could list, and each one has great benefit and a few elements that cause me to pause. Read through the eyes of wisdom and curiosity.
15. Jeremiah 6:16, NIV.

15. THE SAGE'S BOY: BRINGING HIM HOME

1. Laura Hackett Park, "Shalom" (Arrowhead Music Publishing, 2021).
2. Madeleine L'Engle, *A Circle of Quiet* (New York: Crosswicks, Ltd., 1972), 199.
3. Rohr, *Falling Upward*, loc. 509 of 3008, Kindle.
4. NASB.
5. Rohr, *Falling Upward*, 131 and 127 respectively.
6. Eugene Peterson, *The Message* (Colorado Springs, CO: NavPress, 2018); italics added.
7. See Matthew 5:21-30.
8. Check out the Brotherhood Primer and the Brotherhood experiences through Restoration Project. https://www.restorationproject.net/brotherhood.
9. See Colossians 1:15-17.
10. Benner, *The Gift of Being Yourself*, 50.
11. For more on the work we do in the realm of ReStory™ go to https://www.restory.life.
12. Matthew 6: 9-10, NIV.

CONCLUSION

1. Stephen Lawhead, *Pendragon Cycle* (Wheaton, IL: Crossway, 1987).
2. Matthew 18:1-5, NIV; italics added.
3. O'Donohue, *To Bless the Space Between Us*, 71.

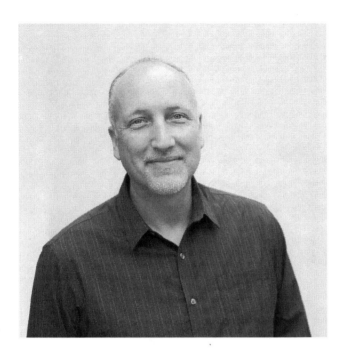

Chris Bruno received a Master of arts in speech from Northwestern University and a Master of arts in counseling psychology from The Seattle School of Theology and Psychology. He is the co-founder and CEO of Restoration Project, a ministry devoted to helping men recover their hearts by healing their wounds, knowing God, and restoring the world. He is a licensed professional counselor, and the founder and CEO of ReStory® Counseling, leading a diverse and collaborative team of storywork counselors around the country. He is the author of *Man Maker Project*, *Brotherhood Primer,* and *Sage*.

Chris has been married to Beth for 27 years and they have three mostly adult children. After spending the better part of a decade in missions in the Near East, they settled in his home state of Colorado. But their love for travel permeates their home and dinnertime conversations and a good adventure is always in the works.

RESTORATION PROJECT

Imagine a world where the inner wounds of men are healed, where men know God deeply and wildly, and where men move from an inner core of strength to restore God's Kingdom in the world around them.

We offer resources and expeditions to help you become more competent and confident as an intentional Son, Brother, and Father.

WWW.RESTORATIONPROJECT.NET

Our Basecamp Boys and Girls, and our Back Country Boys and Girls Expeditions will one of the highlights of your child's lives. Join us this summer! www.RestorationProject.net/Experiences

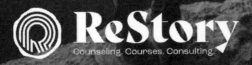

1
FIRST CHAPTER OF BROTHERHOOD PRIMER

This morning I woke up lonely. Not the kind of lonely where I'm convinced I don't have any friends. This kind of lonely feels like an ache in my gut telling me something is amiss. It's not an ache that tells me to lie down for a while or take a Tums. No, this is something far deeper, far closer to the core of who I am, what I'm about, and what it means for me to live the life God gave me. Something that is far more like a haunting than acid reflux.

This something is at the very center of every man's heart.[1] For some guys, even that word feels loaded—*heart*. It's come to mean that amorphous, touchy-feely thing that our post-modern, post-church society has robbed of all real grit. Whether you live in the inner city of Chicago, along the banks of the Mississippi, on Wall Street, on a houseboat in Seattle, or in the vastness of Wyoming, you still have it. Call it what you will—heart, gut, soul, being, center, life, core. They all mean the same thing, really. Let's just say that there's something there that aches. But for what?

If we're honest, it's an ache for other men. It took me several minutes to write that last sentence because it feels so weird to say out loud. We live in a culture that has ultimately demolished the notion of male-male relationship—either hyper-sexualizing it or completely belittling it (think *I Love You, Man*,[2] or the new term "man-date")—that we have lost any true sense of what it means to be close to another guy. The reality is, though, at the core of our beings as men is a hunger and need for other men.

We know it.

We feel it.

But we have lost the art of living as brothers.

And so we give in and settle for the relational table scraps of man-caves, touchdowns, Saturday morning church breakfasts, and over-the-fence backyard conversations, and we completely miss what God intended when he made men to be part of a "brotherhood."

THE LAST SAUSAGE

Over the past 35 years, there has been a resurgence of interest in "man" things—masculinity, manhood, manliness, and what it means to "be a man" in the 21st century. Hundreds of sacred *and* secular organizations have sprung up to help guys "find themselves" in a variety of ways. The man-shelf at the bookstore grew exponentially over these decades, and a growing number of retreats, experiences, and offerings now provides men with more options to develop their masculine hearts. It is a good thing.

Many of these resources have been monumental in the lives of men. They have redirected wayward men, healed broken men, given hope to hopeless men, and restored shattered men. Some online content creators have set out to educate men in the art of being a man, including how to shave, dress, grout tile, sharpen knives, and skip a stone. We honestly can't complain about what good has come from the man-related industry as of late. These books, resources, and retreats have challenged us to do more than merely exist; they've given us a vision for what we could be.

But what about the ache? It's still there.

I was alone on an international flight recently with 16 hours to kill, a private television screen a mere 8 inches from my face, and an arsenal of movie selections at my fingertips. There are several films I would not watch at home with my wife simply because she does not like the war-themed plots or the gruesome battle scenes. It's fine. We watch other things. But if I'm honest, that's not the only reason I like these movies. Usually, in the foxholes and trenches of these epic tales, we find a brotherhood of men who battle together for a common cause. A deep camaraderie forms as they fight darkness, and while the film directors utilize the gruesome and the gory to cloak the deeper narrative, I believe men actually watch these movies for the bond rather than the battle. So, with hours and hours to kill on the flight, I settled in to absorb the unfolding brotherhood on screen.

I watched. I laughed. And I cried. Rather loudly, in fact, in the middle of the night at 35,000 feet over Greenland. I'm sure the woman in the burka a few seats over wondered what the flight attendant put in my drink.[3]

But then we landed, and I moved on.

Of course I did. When a man experiences something moving while he is alone, he shrugs it off or shuts it down and carries on. On the plane I experienced these courageous men in isolation, and as I emerged from the microcosm my headphones and seat 24C produced, I brushed off the emotion and stepped back into "reality." Who has friends like that anyway?

It's the same in the church. We are inundated with information. There is no lack of quality content readily available to us in a thousand different forms. From online sermons to podcasts, from inspirational speakers to seminary programs, from ebooks and Kindle to shelves and shelves of books at the store, we have more Christian information than we can possibly consume. And yet, transformation does not come from information. Transformation results from transformative relationships. And *that* is what this Brotherhood journey is all about.

The reality is that while we have a thousand resources to aid our hearts (or souls, or whatever you call it), a thousand movies to inspire us, a thousand men's breakfasts with a thousand speakers with predictable prayers, we simply move on. Yes, we might remember inklings, but like the smoke from a newly shot rifle, it dissipates the moment the wind blows through.

IT'S ABOUT THE BUTTS

So then, what do we do? Is this what it means to be a man? Is this feeling of loneliness and lostness and dissipation the essence of my existence? Is this book just one more for the man-shelf?

Maybe.

In 2001, my wife and I bought new couches. It was a big deal. We had a baby, and the government decided we deserved an extra tax credit. So we cashed the check, passed "go," and hurried down to the furniture store. Married for six years[4] and in ministry, we'd never actually bought furniture at a store like real adults. Our little Michigan bungalow could barely hold the massive green couches the delivery truck left on our front porch. We would walk in the front door directly into the living room, and there they were. Couches everywhere. It was a bit much.

We kept those same couches for 12 years, 2 countries, 3 states, 5 homes, and 1 re-stuffing. We loved them. But the day came when we needed to say goodbye. Believe it or not, it felt like we were losing a part of our family, and we actually had a ceremony to commemorate their departure from our home.

What I realized about the couches is that they held *story*. The number of butts that sat on them is staggering. The gatherings, the tears, the laughter, the conflicts, the joys, the hard conversations, and even the empty conversations...all had meaning because of *who* the butts belonged to. Those butts belonged to people, and people have stories, and stories are what shape us all. You see, story is the currency of relationship.

I don't remember all of what was said, what was studied, what was learned, or what was revealed. But I do remember the companions along the journey called my life. Every single one of them. Life, real life, has little to do with content or information and far more to do with the narratives that shape and surround us. Connection to others, the kind of connection that attempts to take away the ache, happens when stories are told and held.

In *Tattoos on the Heart*,[5] Gregory Boyle quotes an African proverb that gives clarity to what *Brotherhood Primer* is all about: "A person becomes a person through other people."

Our *becoming* happens through other people.

And the people who have shaped me most have sat with me in the places where stories are shared. Not just "tell me about your vacation" types of stories, but the stories of victory and defeat, of pain and sorrow combined with relief and joy, of hope and fear and courage and terror. These are the stories and these are the relationships in which we are formed.

Half the butts on my couches through the years have belonged to valiant and beautiful women who have offered themselves with such stunning radiance that I can barely imagine life without their color. But this book is not about them or for them.

The other half have belonged to men. In my own life, and in the lives of hundreds of men whose butts have used my chairs, I see an even greater clarification of the African saying. If I may be so bold to modify ancient wisdom, I'd rephrase it to say: "A man becomes a man through other men." Like wet cement that is shaped and molded, I am convinced men become men by the presence and shaping of other men.

That is the ache. To become a man through other men requires other men, yet it takes intentional work for men to get there with each other. And then we get back into that whole weirdness thing, or we make attempts to be in the lives of other men and it just becomes about sin management and accountability, which is so much less than what God's design was ever meant to be. Or we may even have a season of great learning and openness, but we lose it when the winds change. As a result, we come to live with the ache like an old sports injury. We just assume it's part of life.

BROTHERHOOD

But it's not. It's not meant to be part of life. That was never God's intent for men.

The word "brother" means far more than being born from the same parents.[6] To have a brother means you have a companion, a kinsman, an ally, a friend, of the same tribe and of the same purpose. To have a brother means you have a fellow journeyman through this life to shape and to sharpen, to witness each other's peaks and valleys, to disrupt you when you need disrupting, and to carry you when you can't make it on your own.

Brotherhood is another word for a man's becoming.

Brotherhood is synonymous to the holding of story and history in such a way that removes isolation, creates a context for connection, and allows men to enter one another's worlds without judgment, comparison, or competition. Brotherhood's focus is not on the content to be learned or the proper exegesis of a passage or on conformity to a certain ideology. Brotherhood's purpose is to know and be known by other men. For men to be "brothers," they know one another's depravity but hold fiercely and tightly to one another's glory in order to see each other become the men God intended for them to be. A brother is an ally of the Father on your behalf.

BROTHERHOOD AND THE BIBLE

There is something about togetherness that God seems to enjoy. As a Triune God, where relationship is perfected between the Father, Son, and Spirit, He designed His image bearers on earth to know and experience companionship. Aloneness is antithetical to God's design.

The Bible is full of stories about brothers. And to be honest, their track record for having positive relationships isn't too good. Famous Bible brothers include Cain and Abel, Jacob and Esau, James and John (otherwise known as the "Sons of Thunder"), Joseph and his unhappy eleven brothers, and even Jesus's parable of the two brothers, to name but a few. Many of the brothers in the scriptures turn out to be archenemies. But I'm not talking about blood brothers who share DNA. I'm talking about *brotherhood*. Biological brothers are in relationship because they share parental origins. They had no choice in their earthly connection. But men choose to participate in brotherhood.

When we make this shift in understanding from *brothers* to *brotherhood*, we see a plethora of fantastic examples in the scriptures as well. Some of the most notable are David and Jonathan, Elijah and Elisha, Paul and Barnabas, Jesus and Peter, and James and John. Men choose to participate in brotherhood relationships out of an inherent need to be with other men. God did not design men to live in isolation.[7]

Consider even the incarnation of Jesus—the Son descending from heaven, taking on human flesh as a man, and coming to live on earth amongst his creation. The name "Emmanuel" means "God *with* us" and is a powerful reminder that God's heart for togetherness compels Him to step into human history in order to be our brother and friend. How is it that the God of all creation chose to walk amongst us? Even more stunning is the fact that He chose for Himself a brotherhood of men! Despite His participation in the Godhead, Jesus still wanted and needed to be surrounded by a close-knit group of other guys. Not because He had to, but because He chose to. He says, "I no longer call you servants....Instead, I have called you *friends*."[8]

If Jesus did it, then I supposed we should as well.

Brotherhood, in the end, is about being *with*. With is very different than "next to" or "doing the same activity." No, true *withness* is about entering into one another's lives in the places and ways that matter. *That* is the choice and motivation of brotherhood.

THE ULTIMATE GOAL

I recently read a book about a completely different topic.[9] In it, the author made reference to some of the primary findings from men involved in the Promise Keepers' movement in the 1990s. The number one common thread of pain and loss among men: friendlessness. Number two: emotional isolation from other men. Number three: confusion about masculinity in the current cultural context. The list goes on and confirms over and over again the extreme need for men to relearn male-male relationality. We need it. We are desperate for it.

And yet the challenge is this: though we are lonely and isolated men, we do not have a roadmap to connecting with other men. Many of us were never taught how to step past the superficial into actual masculine relationships, having witnessed the anemic friendships of our fathers or experienced for ourselves the "man code" that discourages deeper emotional connection with other guys. Ultimately, my hope is that through the process laid out in *Brotherhood Primer* you will come a few steps closer to knowing and experiencing brotherhood with other men. I also believe God desires for all men to be part of an authentic brotherhood, and it is in this belief that I rest, knowing that hope can be a dangerous spark to ignite a powerful fire.

NUTS AND BOLTS: HOW THIS WORKS

But this is not a book. It's a "primer." It's not designed to be a book that you read and think about by yourself in your quiet time, and then put away and move on. It's meant to prime the pump not just of your thinking, but of your actual brotherhood relationships. You can read all you want about becoming a brother, but until you *do it*–

engage other men's hearts; sit across from them and have that awkward moment of "I don't know what to do or say or think"; actually *do* brotherhood–it won't change a thing about you.

Remember, information does not change people. Relationships do. What I have provided here is meant to be a scaffolding and a catalyst to relationship. The most important content you bring to any brotherhood is not this book or anything I have to say. No, the most important content you can bring to other men is your own self with your own stories. *That* is the primary text.

Yes, you can read this book alone, but it is designed for you to engage alongside a small brotherhood of men. There are parts for you to consider alone, write down your thoughts, and reflect on your own life. However, the real grit and growth will occur as you take these reflections and offer them in trust to the other men you've gathered.

The first important step is to gather a group of men. These can be men you've known for a long time or men you met just last week. The important element is that these guys must have some desire for something more in their lives, both as individuals and, more importantly, in their relationships with other men. I recommend a group of 4 to 6 men. Any more, and it is easily sidetracked; any less, and it's just plain weird.

What are you asking them to do? This is a 10- to 16-week[10] primer designed to facilitate further personal exploration into what God is doing in your own manhood as well as to bring other men into authentic contact with your soul. This is <u>not</u> an "accountability" group. It is <u>not</u> a "Bible study" or a "men's group." This is a different animal. In essence, you are asking these guys to address the lack of depth in their current male-male friendships by seeking out more of God's design for life together with brothers along the way. Consider it an experiment.

Practically, you are asking them to walk through this primer with you, engaging their own stories and their own hearts along the way, while seeing what may develop between you as brothers. You are asking them to commit to reading the chapters, engaging the questions, and meeting together once a week.[11] Each week's Brotherhood gathering should be about an hour and a half. Start by doing one chapter per week. Then, when prompted, set aside several weeks for each man to share his story (much more detail on what that looks like in the upcoming chapters). After you finish this journey, it's up to you how you proceed. Again, this is designed to prime the pump, not be the pump.

While many guys like to gather at a restaurant or pub, I'd suggest avoiding those kinds of places for these meetings. It's just too loud and distracting, and you may be having conversations that you won't want overheard. Find a garage, basement, or backyard fire pit. I share more thoughts about the importance of this space in future chapters. For now, trust me.

Now I realize the bar is set pretty high. The greatest commodity for most men is their time. It's a lot to ask, but I am not going to apologize. The reality is we spend time, money, and energy on those things that are most valuable to us. Think about your commitment to the gym, to your career, to watching the evening news. You do it because you want it. You do it because it's important. There are plenty of barriers that prevent men from engaging in this kind of process with one another, the foremost likely being time. But I've kept the bar high because true brotherhood, when lived out over a lifetime, takes time and commitment. It's just a fact. If I lowered the bar, I'd be selling you a generic set of goods and training you to swim in the kiddie pool rather than setting your sights on the Olympic gold.

The reality is that each group will have a life of its own. God created each of you to participate in your own way and at this time of your life. Never before in history and never again will the uniqueness of your group occur. It's wonderful and curious and worthy of notice. The only thing you can control is the length of time you meet and how engaged you will be when you meet. Ultimately, it's up to you, your comrades, and the Spirit of God.

GATHERING YOUR BROTHERHOOD

Probably the hardest part of this whole thing is gathering a group of guys to do this with you. You may already have a few in mind. You may be thumbing through your contact list hoping for a name or two to jump out at you. Either way, asking another guy to be involved in this kind of thing is nerve-racking. It just is.

First, pray. Ask God for direction in who to ask. Who are the men He's wanting you to pursue? I am convinced this is God's design for men. As a result, I believe it is His desire to provide every man with other men with whom to journey through this life. He's not holding out on you. Ask Him. Listen. Then ask them.

Second, have a "start date." Although the material starts off with content, I believe the best place to start with men is *play*. Invite the guys to some sort of gathering where you've got some good fun planned. Maybe it's a Scotch night around the fire pit. Maybe it's a poker night. Maybe it's a day of waterskiing on the lake. Maybe it's a hike or a shooting range. It doesn't matter as long as there is some sort of "intro" activity that gets the guys doing things together. It's vital to have a basis of relationship before diving into the categories of the heart. Your group may have a long history together, or you may be complete strangers. Either way, play is an essential place to start. Just think of it as loosening up the soil for the deeper things to come.

Third, discuss your commitment to the process at this initial gathering. It would be better to opt out before starting than to get involved and then have to back out in the middle. Can everyone create time to meet consistently and complete the individual work? We are all busy, and this primer requires a serious level of commitment—not to the primer, but to the other men in the group. Is every man willing to make sacrifices? Will everyone be at every gathering for the next 10 to 16 weeks? If not, can schedule modifications be made to accommodate?

Additionally, the primer will ask men to go to places personally and relationally they may be fearful and reticent to go. Is everyone willing to jump off that cliff, believing there is something more, something better? It is just plain awkward to be gathered with guys sharing their hearts and perspectives while one or two remain silent or distant. Will you be willing to step into the ring? Will you allow yourself to be challenged by the other men when they see you hiding in the bushes?

I have provided you with a **BROTHERHOOD COVENANT** and **RULES OF ENGAGEMENT** in the following pages. (You can also download the free pdf version at restorationproject.net/brotherhood. I highly recommend each man in the group to get his own copy.). The purpose is to formally agree together that you are committed to this process. I have found that men respond to a specific call. Rallying together around these basic agreements and covenants is a vital beginning to the shaping of your Brotherhood group.

Fourth, get the buy-in of your wife or significant other. If the guys are married or in a romantic relationship, it's important for their wives/girlfriends to be on board with this process. In one sense, these upcoming months will require time, energy, emotion, and focus from each man—meaning that he has to take this from somewhere. Ask each man to speak with his wife/girlfriend about what this could mean for him, for them, and for her. I am convinced that when men are *true men* as God intended, everyone benefits. The last thing a guy wants is to commit to a process like this and then have his wife/girlfriend either not understand, resent it, or undermine it in some way. Her buy-in is crucial.

Fifth, commit to an end. This is a 10- to 16-week primer. When will it be over? My goal is to help create relationships that will far outlive this process. However, at the end of the primer, it is best to reevaluate the relationships that have been built and give guys the "opt-out" option. Having that freedom of choice allows guys to dive more deeply into the process and avoid the feeling of being locked in for a lifetime.

Sixth, each man will need his own copy of *Brotherhood Primer*. Before the group's first gathering, make sure everyone has ample time to wander through the chapter titles, rhythms, and commitments.

And finally, start. Pray, pray, pray. Ask, ask, ask. Play, and then begin.

A NOTE ON FACILITATING THE BROTHERHOOD

If you are the man giving leadership to this group, let me start by commending you. Well done. You have made a brave and bold step, one that I believe will cause goodness to ripple through the lives of families and communities for generations to come. I imagine the decision to start this journey comes out of both desire and past discouragement. By stepping into the ring, you are actively defying isolation, loneliness, and passivity. Thank you.

I've already said it, but I'll say it again. This is a different animal. Many of you may have experience leading small groups and accountability groups, facilitating meetings, or leading others in general. Your past experience will indeed be meaningful and helpful. Yet there are some significant differences between a typical church small group and what this primer seeks to achieve.

Ultimately, the key for the leader is to remember that the content provided in this book is far less important than the stories shared and the relationships built. There is no need to get all the questions asked and answered and no need to argue about the perspectives written. Of primary importance is how the individual men interact with their experience of being a man. My goal has been to provide a springboard for discussion, not to write "the absolute right way of being a man." Many will have different perspectives. Some will outright disagree with what I've written or proposed. As the facilitator, it is your role to make sure that the focus of the conversation during the gatherings is less about parsing words or making declarative, universal statements about manhood and more about *what we* as men are learning about manhood from one another. Remember, "men become men through other men."

Therefore, I've called it a "primer" for a reason: to prime the pump to get things flowing. The point is not the prime. The point is the well and the unique outflow that gets going as a result. Yes, there will be times when the facilitator will need to reorient and refocus the group toward the goal. But that goal is not the same as most content-based groups. The goal is to know and be known, not focus on the questions or the material.

The goal is to know and be known, not focus on the questions or the material.

If you have chosen to gather and facilitate a group, I commend you for your courage, your tenacity, and your commitment both to your own soul as well as to the well-being of others. Maybe you are operating out of desperation. Maybe it's vision.

In the end, they are the same thing.

QUESTIONS AS YOU BEGIN

Who will you gather? Write the names of the men you want to invite to be part of the Brotherhood. Aim for 4 to 6 men. No more than 6, no less than 4.

What day will your Brotherhood gather? What time? Where?

What will you do for your initial time together to get to know one another and have some fun?

What day will you all need to start reading/reflecting on the primer material in order to be ready for the first gathering?

BROTHERHOOD COVENANT

A covenant is an agreement and commitment, a promise. For the Brotherhood process to be effective, all men need to be either fully in or fully out. Not in between. This is a rigorous process, and it is best for everyone to agree that he is *all in* before you begin. It's not signing your life away or making a long-term commitment to be part of the group beyond these 10 to 16 weeks, but it is stepping forward and making a promise that you will make the effort to fully participate in the process.

The men in this Brotherhood group include (maximum of 6 men):

Our Brotherhood gatherings will occur at _ am/pm at the following location:

We have agreed to meet on the following dates:

Confidentiality is an essential element to the development of any close relationship. You will be asked to investigate parts of your life and story as a man and to bring these reflections authentically to the others in your Brotherhood. You will not be coerced to share but challenged to go to new places in your own life and story, as well as in your relationships with other men. You agree to honor yourself and the other men by holding what is shared in this group in confidence. Confidence, or *con-fide,* means to have "faith with" others.

By signing below, I covenant with these men to complete the individual questions for each chapter, attend all gatherings, hold confidence, uphold the rules of engagement, and participate with as much authenticity as I can muster.

I have spoken with my wife or significant other, and she both understands the importance of this in my life and supports me as I pursue God's fullness for me in brotherhood with other men.

Signed:

RULES OF ENGAGEMENT:

In order for this Brotherhood to work, we need to establish some basic Rules of Engagement. These are essential agreements that will help us stay on course and create an atmosphere that is safe, inviting, and encouraging. (Go to restorationproject.net/brotherhood to download this document for everyone to sign.)

NO FIXING | The intention of this type of group is to provide an environment where we do not seek to "fix" each other. A man needs the freedom to say what is on his mind and heart without the fear that others will want to placate, advise, or offer insight into what he should do. Everyone needs to agree to listen and not fix. Advice kills story. The only time advice is to be offered is if it is specifically invited.

TIME IS CRUCIAL | Time is one of men's most valuable assets. It is vitally important to respect one another's time. This means showing up on time and ending on time. If you would like to have additional time, go ahead...as long as it is agreed upon by all.

STAY PRESENT | You are in this to learn from and connect with one another. Therefore, you must all agree to engage one another from a place of curiosity rather than assumption. Additionally, it is important to stay engaged with the one talking rather than allow yourself to daydream or anticipate what you will say next. The ache men often feel is to know that others are truly "with" them when they are talking, not drifting away or jockeying for the next comment. Listen. Stay.

SUSPEND JUDGMENT | As this group gets going, you will likely encounter a variety of thoughts, lifestyles, opinions, theologies, and preferences that are vastly different from your own. This is not a place to correct or corral other men. It is, however, a place for you to consider other perspectives, other stories, and other ways of being. If you disagree with someone else's thoughts or choices, this is not the place to voice your concerns. This is a brotherhood, not a thought-police conference.

RIGHTS AND WRONGS | In order for an atmosphere of safety to be established, every man has the right to "pass" at any point. If he chooses to do so, the group should not push him. The only thing the group may ask is, "why?" It is wrong to force someone to talk about something that is too raw or vulnerable if he does not feel ready. It is better to stay in the group than to feel alienated and leave because of boundary violations.

SHOW UP | You will likely have to fight the urge to abandon the whole thing. Something may come up inside of you that does not want to take the risk to share. Shadows of fight or flight. Or maybe you will find yourself suddenly too tired to focus and engage. Or maybe you feel like what you shared was too much or too little and the other guys think you are an idiot. The most vital part of building relationships with other guys is consistently showing up and acknowledging those thoughts to them. In fact, one of the most transformational ways to deepen relationship with other men is to talk about how it feels to be in relationship with them. Share about your fears, your hopes, your anxieties, your shame. It will open the door to something far deeper than your silence ever could.

PERSONAL REFLECTION

- First, go to RestorationProject.net/BrotherhoodQuiz and take the five-minute quiz to see what some of your core motivations are for saying "yes" to this group. The more you can understand your own desires and vision for this journey, and the more you share those with the men, the more likely it will be that you get what you came for. The results will be automatically emailed to you. Bring that email with you to the next group. The fact is, the results are secondary to the conversation that ensues as you collectively discuss your hopes for this gathering. Prior to that, spend a few minutes reflecting on these questions:

- How did those results land for you? What surprised you?
- In what way were you, or were you not, aware of your desires for this group?
- Why do you imagine the other men said "yes" to Brotherhood?
- Is there anything else you'd like to share with the men about your vision for this journey?

GROUP DISCUSSION

- How did this introductory chapter hit you? What did you notice?
- What did you think about the results of the quiz? (If the men haven't taken the quiz, take five minutes and have the guys do the quiz.) How did you feel when you got your results?
- What were your results?
- As you read the Rules of Engagement, what are your thoughts? What excites you? What feels intimidating?
- Overall, how are you feeling about the process of going through this primer? Are you all in?
- (Take time, if you haven't already, to get schedules aligned and decide where you'll meet.)
- Pray for the coming weeks, for each other, and for yourselves.